BABY BOOMER LONGEVITY

strategies to transform your health

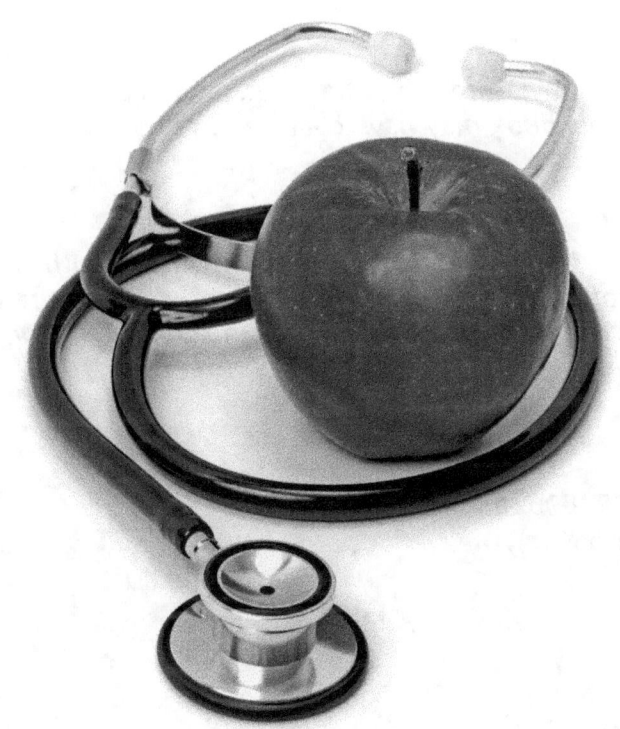

PAUL DAVIS MD

Baby Boomer Longevity: Strategies to Transform Your Health is available in both soft copy and eBook editions and can be purchased online at amazon.com, barnesandnoble.com and booksamillion.com. You can also request your local bookstore to order a copy.

ISBN-13: 978-1479281626
ISBN-10: 147928162X

DEDICATION

*T*his book is dedicated to all those individuals in my life, who helped me recognize the "healer within us" and the ways in which to use our innate gifts to help others attain perfect health.

In particular, I dedicate this book to my mother who unfailingly encouraged me to proceed through many adversities to attain my inner desire of being a good physician and healer.

Her strong will guided many an individual in their chosen fields. I was fortunate as her son to have her 86 years of encouragement on my side.

This book is dedicated to the healer within you, the reader, in the hopes that it will assist you in healing not only yourself, but also those around you.

HEALTH BOOK CONCEPT

To help readers understand medical-health concepts that they can apply to facilitate individual healing and quality of life applications, with an awareness of mind-body-spirit connections and alternative health methodologies -- along with traditional allopathic medicine.

TABLE OF CONTENTS

Chapter 1 TRANSFORMING YOUR HEALTH 1

    Medical Methodology...3

    Attaining Longevity..4

Chapter 2 THE BASIC THEORY 5

    Our Food Chain 6

    A Healthy Lifestyle 10

    Treat the Body Right 12

Chapter 3 COMPLIMENTARY THERAPIES 13

    East Meets West..13

    Aromatherapy...17

    Homeopathy 18

    Reiki 21

    Shiatsu..22

    What the Bible Says About Healthy Living 31

    Meditation 32

    Rejuvenation...38

Chapter 4 THE PROCESS OF AGING...............................40

    When the Body Ages 43

    Changes to Our Senses 44

    Medications 47

    Antioxidants and Their Role in Aging 50

    When Our Muscles Hurt 51

    Smoother Skin, Fewer Wrinkles 54

    The Aging Brain 57

Chapter 5 MEDICAL CONDITIONS 65

Arthritis... 66

Fibromyalgia 69

Chronic Fatigue 69

Sleep Disorders 73

Depression 73

Stress 74

Hypoglycemia... 74

Gallstones 77

Constipation.. 78

ADHD Attention Deficit Hyperactivity Disorder 80

Alzheimer's Disease 82

Liver Disease 84

Allergies 88

Motion Sickness 92

Tattoos and Piercing Infection Risks................................ 94

Mosquito Borne Disease 96

Travel Tips – Staying Healthy... 103

Heat Illness and Dehydration: Protecting Yourselves 104

Surgical Healing 107

Therapeutic Massage.. 109

Chapter 6 CANCER PREVENTION.. 115

Cancer Statistics... 115

The Cancer Prevention Food List 117

Reducing Stress When Fighting Cancer............................ 120

Chapter 7 HEART HEALTH... 121

Heart Disease 121

Heart Testing 129

Natriuretic Peptides 131

Chapter 8 METABOLIC SYNDROME 133

Metabolic Risk Factors 133

Outlook 134

Chapter 9 FERTILITY 135

Male Fertility Health 135

Female Fertility Health 137

Chapter 10 FLU SHOTS 139

When to Get Vaccinated 139

Where to Get Vaccinated 140

Who Should Get Vaccinated 140

Tips for Preventing the Flu 143

Chapter 11 FAITH HEALING 147

The Role of Faith in Healing 148

My Healer Study 151

Transformational Medicine 153

Chapter 12 THE ROLE OF FOOD IN HEALTHY LIVING 173

Good Fat Bad Fat 154

Preserving Skin 161

Free Radicals 162

Healing Foods 162

You Are What You Eat – The Healthy Vegan Diet 170

The Truth About Eating Red Meat 174

Nuts and Their Nutritive Value 179

Net Carbs and Artificial Sweeteners 183

Positive Nutrition 185

Chapter 13 HERBS VITAMINS & SUPPLEMENTS 189

Nutritional Supplementation Against Stress 189

Useful Healing Herbs 191

    Flower Remedies 196

Chapter 14 A LOOK AT DIETS... 200

The SAD Diet... 200

Simple Strategies to Healthier Eating.................................... 201

Diets and Diabetes 204

A Case Against Very Low Calorie Diets 206

A Sensible Diet 209

Dr. Davis's Sensible Diet 212

Exercise... 215

The American Diet.. 216

Biblical Diet – The Maker's Diet 218

Bland Diet.. 220

Japanese Diet 221

The Chinese Diet.. 226

Mediterranean Diet.. 230

The Portfolio Diet: Lowers Cholesterol 231

Body for Life Diet 234

Ornish Diet... 236

Vegetarian Diet 240

Heart Disease Diet.. 242

Stroke and Diabetes Diet.. 244

French Diet... 244

Eating Well for Optimum Health – The Weil's Approach.............. 248

Chapter 15 FAST FOOD DANGERS 251

Chapter 16 WEIGHT LOSS 257

The New Weight Loss 257

Healthy Weight Loss 266

Thallotherapy and Losing Weight................................277

Chapter 17 HUMAN PERFORMANCE AFFECTED BY

DEHYDRATION..288

Chapter 18 DELICIOUS HEALTHY RECIPES 291

Beverages and Hors d'Ouevres 291

Sauces, Gravy, Chutney & Relish 303

Entres 304

INTRODUCTION

Welcome to the new world of medicine where healing and transforming your health are a joint effort between you and your health care providers. Through my years of medical training I have seen a great deal of changes in allopathic medicine. In this book, I will incorporate those changes in advice to the reader.

If I had lived this life in Western Europe's Middle Ages I also would have seen a significant number of changes in the healing arts. Similarly, if I had lived in the age of Buddha, I would have seen a guru from India having changed a great deal of the treatments, which my fellow humans would have received.

From a medical point of view, one can go through history, and see how health has affected both how we live, and how we die. Epidemics combined with poor treatment techniques have seen the rise and fall of many governments. Medical phenomena have aided the acceptance of certain religious beliefs, often times called miracles.

A university professor, Ludwig von Bertalanffy, who taught an innocuous course called "History of Medicine", inspired my interest in a more holistic approach to medical science. Professor Bertalanffy, the originator of Systems Approach, was very adept at stimulating our young minds to thinking beyond the box from a medical point of view.

Although, I come from several generations of medical practitioners, I was never forced into becoming a doctor. In fact, my father was an engineer and wanted me to do the same. My father's side-of-the-family were not doctors, but on my mother's side, the family tree traces us back to the Norman invasion of France.

Apparently, a great number of my ancestors were the healers of those infamous invaders, and later of the courts of France. During the French Revolution, all association with the aristocracy was dropped, and the family began a long lineage of professorships at the newly emerging "medical science" in the universities.

So ingrained in our family's history was this healing heritage that even if one didn't want to be a doctor, you had to. My maternal grandfather and one of his older brothers did not want to become doctors. Secretly, they went to engineering school, in addition to medical school, and became qualified in both professions. Something we would have trouble doing in the 21st century!!

Both my grandfather and granduncle came to America during the Gold Rush era and practiced their profession as engineers. They designed bridges, roads, and other infrastructure for the booming West of America. They never personally practiced medicine, but supported many educational institutions, which furthered their healing tradition.

In any event, this is the reason I was raised in the San Francisco Bay area through high school. Following an interest in genetics, I went to the University of Alberta in Edmonton, Alberta, Canada. After completing my Bachelor of Science degree there, I stayed in the Canadian system of medical education finishing my studies on the other side of Canada in Nova Scotia and Newfoundland.

An interlude of graduate studies at the University of Southern California in Los Angeles in physical medicine and rehabilitation changed the otherwise 15-year period of time in Canada.

During various points during those studies, I spent time as a medical volunteer in various parts of the world. A good deal of that was in Central and South America and Southeast Asia. Through all of those experiences, I was able to see medical practices that were unlike those that I had learned in traditional, allopathic medical school and residency. The underlying theme that one could take from all of those experiences was that all forms of medicine worked to a certain extent.

This book is a compilation of many years experience, research, and study in medical sciences. Over the years, I have been a medical director of allopathic medical clinics, hospital departments, corporate medical programs, etc. I've worked in big cities, rural outposts, on ships, and just about any other place a doctor is needed.

In 1978, I started a medical volunteer organization that supplied doctors throughout the world. That organization developed into consulting group that developed medical programs for hospitals, clinics, governments, hotels, and VIPs that wanted a special approach to medical science.

Over the last number of years, we've developed specific medical programs, and housed them in health resorts throughout the world administered by the hotel, or hospital that has requested our services.

These are places where one can go to be treated or rejuvenated in a beautiful, healing environment without leaving the skills of modern western medicine behind.

This book encompasses many of the philosophies and techniques, which I have found to be successful throughout my career as a healer. This is a combination of Western and Eastern philosophies and practices.

It is my belief that this gentler approach treats disease using not only the most recent advances we have in western allopathic medicine, but also incorporating the other healing arts of the world.

Our methodology encourages the body to treat itself and repair mechanisms to be able to fight off future problems–disease, infections, digestive processes, etc. These methods will also allow the body to heal faster from necessary or elective procedures.

This book is aimed at primarily helping my age group – the Baby Boomers, but the theories are universal to all those who want appropriate strategies to transform their health in a positive way.

And on that note – let us begin the journey into a healthier lifestyle.

CHAPTER 1

TRANSFORMING YOUR HEALTH

Many people in this world would like to be free of physical and mental discomforts. Perfect health is defined as a state where a person is physically and mentally free from disease and suffers no pain. Some would add that perfect health includes never growing old or never dying too young. Transforming your health may help you get closer to that lofty goal.

In order to achieve longevity and transform your health one may need to change many aspects of their normal routine. It may take months or years to reverse various poor habits that we have acquired or diseases that need to be treated.

Although we can help as physicians, a great deal of health is dependent upon self-healing and a great deal of hard work on the part of the individual in many cases. Perfect health, incorporates protecting what one already has in a healthy lifestyle and body, while alleviating the various disease disorders that one has acquired.

Diseases are present in our society. Some people get sick, then again some people don't. Our diet, activities, sleep, stress, and our genetic makeups are all factors in whether we have perfect health or not.

For the most part viruses, bacteria, fungi, allergies, deterioration of body parts, cancers, and exposures to various chemicals in our environment cause diseases. Although all of these things are present in our society, not everybody gets sick.

Even if you do get sick with the same disease process as the person next door, you may not have as harmful or severe a disease process as they do. For example: Patient #1 may have a heart attack, and die immediately; whereas Patient #2 may have a heart attack and live a long and prosperous life. Then again, Patient #3 may have a serious heart attack and he/she is assisted by a variety of modern technology, where blood vessels are opened with medication and/or stents. Or, whereas Patient #4 may have a milder heart attack and takes a variety of Ayurvedic, or other natural medicines to more gradually retrain the heart muscle to function normally.

In other words, four people, four heart attacks, and four different outcomes. This applies to all diseases and illnesses, which is also why treating anyone can be difficult sometimes.

Each person has a unique makeup and level of immunity. Immunity is simply the defense that each of us has against disease. Two individuals may harbor the same bacteria. One will get the disease, while the other will get nothing, because the second person has more resistance/immunity.

White blood cells are the main entity that gives us our immunity. They phagocytize (eat) the bacteria or other dangerous organisms and digest them into a product that is non-pathogenic. This is one of our main sources of protection against disease.

So what is Transforming Your Health really about?

✓ Transforming Your Health is part of a global paradigm shift in health care.

✓ Transforming Your Health searches for a healing system that promotes health using natural non-toxic substances when possible.

✓ Transforming Your Health seeks to use the least invasive of modern Western technology when urgent care is required.

✓ Transforming Your Health also recognizes the important role of the mind and emotions in having a perfectly healthy individual.

If you follow the logic behind this new paradigm of Transforming Your Health, one must describe events as possibilities instead of certainties, and recognize the interconnectedness of all phenomena in science.

One must recognize a more holistic view of how events in the human body occur, rather than the old view that often explains events in terms of separate, unrelated components in a human machine.

Medical Methodology

Students used to be taught Anatomy, Physiology, Histology, Pathology, etc. in medical school. Then just as I entered medical school, there was a shift to the 'systems approach'.

The Old View

The old view looked at the human body's machine with separate systems, organs, and tissues that would malfunction individually. The old view of the human machine also separated the mind and the body into separate entities.

The New View

The new method of teaching students and the Transforming Your Health paradigm, acknowledge the mutual interdependence of the physical body, mind, emotions, and the environment in creating health and disease.

This new view of perfect health removes the physician or healer as the absolute authority in the healing process and makes the patient/individual responsible for many of the things that happen.

The Healer Within Us

I firmly believe that, within each of us, there is a healer. Having been raised as a Quaker (Society of Friends), we were taught that there was God in each of us. In the Quaker belief, this was in the form of light, and that this light shone in every person at a different luminosity.

Good people had much more light (God) within them than not so good people. I now personally believe that God, in whatever form one believes he/she exists has given every human grace. How we accept this grace, and go forth with it is paramount to how we deal with our own bodies and the rest of humanity. Progressing this thought process to healing and transforming your health, one can believe that there is some healer in all human beings.

To heal ourselves, we must set this in motion. Many religious and other spiritual belief systems have various modifications on this theme.

For many patients, this is a totally new concept, since previously they have depended upon outside sources, to guide every single aspect of their health and well-being.

My contention with Transforming Your Health, is that physicians and other healers, need to be guides to help the individual awaken the healer within them; and to assist by applying whatever technological, and traditional methodologies are possible to make that person whole and healthy.

Attaining Longevity

In reality, to attain longevity, you need to hook into the healing forces in the universe. Our modern medical allopathic practices, the botanical medicines of homeopathy, Ayurveda, and naturopathy are all tools, which nature has provided.

It is our role as physicians and healers to facilitate and promote the process that nature has in its universal force. We do this through the aid of chemical, natural, physical, spiritual, and mental therapies.

Transforming Your Health is not un-natural. It should actually be the normal state for a human being along with an inner sense of well-being. In this transformation, the body should be clear of toxins; the mind should be at peace with no depression, or other negative emotions; and organs should be functioning in the manner they were intended.

Unfortunately, in our modern world, the physical and mental systems for many individuals do not function perfectly, which causes deterioration in the body working properly. This dysfunction weakens our body systems, opening the door for chronic, degenerative, and non-specific diseases to develop.

These can evolve into serious diseases, such as cancer, heart disease, diabetes, liver failure, degenerative diseases -- such as rheumatoid arthritis -- and many other diseases, ultimately damaging an individual's overall health and wellness.

The goal of Transforming Your Health to attain longevity in a healthy and peaceful way is to reverse these negative effects of daily living and restore the natural state of health and wellness, bringing balance back to the body.

CHAPTER 2

THE BASIC THEORY

When we look at what effects our body, we need to know how we can relate to those things. Our state of health is generally considered a balance between the things that support our body's strengths, and the things that are harmful to our body in general.

Our genetic makeup provides a background for basic elements to interact. The ultimate outcome of this balance is whether we are healthy or sick. If there are harmful elements that attack our body including things we eat, and our genetic makeup is not strong enough to resist these things, our body may fail to ward off other disease processes.

Our natural condition is supposed to be good health with vibrant bodies, bright minds, and the ability to do whatever we want. Unfortunately, this is not the case and many people end up with various ailments.

Our society is now plagued with an epidemic of obesity and various degenerative illnesses. We are seeing middle-aged and baby boomers fall victims to Alzheimer's disease, and various other mental disorders prematurely.

Is it our lifestyle? Is it our environment? Is it our diet? Is it our genetics? Or, as some doomsday soothsayers say, is it because we have "lived a bad life"? If it were the latter, who is to define a perfect life?

Based upon various calculations, the lifespan of a human being at this time, in most developed nations, should be approximately 85 years old. These 85 years should be filled with the ability to move, think, see, hear, and be productive members of society. There is one large group of individuals that actually meet this goal and live active, productive lives in western societies (more about them later in the book).

Why then, are there so many hospitals, nursing homes, mental institutes, supported living institutes, personal support workers, a multibillion dollar pharmaceutical industry, and the inability of many governments to even start to cope with the cost of health care?

Our Food Chain

The old adage " you are what you eat" has never been truer. There is a great deal of evidence, which strongly implicates that the main cause of death and disability in the world today is based upon the diet that most humans eat.

Many forms of cancer, coronary artery disease, obesity, diabetes, and various other chronic diseases can be linked to the diets we eat.

Many will say that they have known individuals deep in their 90s, who have smoked all their life, consumed large amounts of alcohol daily, eaten fried, greasy animal food based diets, and never exercised.

Obviously, this is in defense of various lifestyles of the individuals who point to these 90-year-olds, that they would like to continue themselves. Many years ago, we did not have the same environment that we currently live in.

Most of our food is not grown or raised on soil that is rich in the nutrients our bodies need. Various chemicals from the industry surrounding the agricultural fields pollute much of that soil. Innumerable additives are placed in our food, which can eliminate the goodness of the food itself and put the recipient at risk from various carcinogens.

Many of these additives are in our food to allow greater marketability, longevity on shelves, and profitability. Similarly, the air we breathe and the water we drink, are far from similar to those the 90-year-old was exposed to, when he or she was young.

Add to the physical issues various issues with stress that our modern society has developed for us and you have only a few of the many reasons why the argument that some use for their current lifestyle holds no water.

Almost all the diseases that we currently suffer from stem from various aspects of our environment, and a great deal of that environment is in contact with food in one way or another.

If you don't take care of your body, where are you going to live?

How to Stay Healthy

- Healthy habits affect your overall health. Cancer, stroke, heart disease, diabetes, along with other serious illnesses, can <u>all</u> be prevented, at least partially, by making good healthy lifestyle choices.

- Don't smoke. The use of tobacco leads to 440,000 deaths in the US annually. Tobacco is the number one cause of illnesses like lung cancer, heart disease, emphysema, mouth cancer, bladder cancer, and throat cancer. So quit smoking today.

- Try to limit your alcohol intake to occasional drinks on the weekend or a special party, or better still, none. At maximum, limit your alcohol intake to no more than 1 drink a day for both women and men. 1 can of beer, a 1-ounce jigger of spirits, or a 3-ounce glass of wine are all equal to 1 drink. Too much alcohol can cause liver damage, liver cancer, Alzheimer's, etc. The much-publicized 'positive benefits of red wine' comes from the grape seed and only 1-tablespoon a day of red wine produces the 'benefits'-- not the whole bottle.

- If you are overweight, lose the extra weight. Extra weight is responsible for diabetes, high cholesterol, high blood pressure, certain cancers, stroke, gallbladder, and arthritis in weight bearing joints.

- Exercise. It can help to prevent osteoporosis, depression, high blood pressure, heart disease, stroke, back injury, and it can play a role in colon cancer. Try to exercises for a minimum of 30 minutes a day for a minimum of 4 days a week. However, any exercise is better than no exercise at all.

- Don't use tanning booths (some Canadian provinces have now outlawed tanning booths for teenagers), and don't sunbathe. Sun exposure is directly linked to skin cancer as well as other types of cancer, and wrinkled skin. Use sunscreen of at least SPF 45. Get your Vitamin D from a simple pill.

- Practice safe sex to avoid STD's (sexually transmitted diseases). Use condoms and a spermicidal (to kill sperm).

- Keep vaccinations up to date: Tetanus–diphtheria booster every 10 years, annual flu shots, travel vaccines, etc. If you are a prostitute, take them all.

- Check your breasts. Breast cancer is the second most common cause of death for women. Have a baseline mammogram. Then every two years from the age of 40, and after 50, it should be annual. (These guidelines change regularly and depending on your insurance or the country in which you live).

- Get a regular Pap smear. A Pap smear should be done within three years of becoming sexually active or by the age of 21. It should be done every five years until age 40, then annually unless your doctor or health plan says otherwise. A Pap smear should be done up on this schedule until the age of 65, then your doctor will probably recommend less frequently, even if you have had a hysterectomy.

- Have a yearly physical and discuss risk factors with your doctor.

- Ask your doctor about cancer screening like fecal occult blood screening.

- Check your blood pressure regularly and keep it within lower limits.

- Realize that the present moment is all you ever have. Make the *Now* the primary focus of your life. You may pay brief visits to the past and future, when required to deal with the practical aspects of your life situation, but always say "yes" to the present moment. Surrender to what is. Say "yes" to life -- and see how life suddenly starts working for you rather than against you.

- Remember this always: nothing that we ever did or that has been done to us can touch or destroy the radiant essence of who we are. When we surrender to that Being, to that which is and become fully present to the *Now* the past ceases to have any power. We do not need it anymore.

How to Have Vital Health Now

Some vital nutrients are necessary for good health and life extension. These same nutrients can also help you to lose weight. When trying to lose weight, most people focus on the number of calories they eat.

However, if you eat a low-calorie diet, which is low in nutrients, it is as bad for your health as if you were eating a diet that was high in calories and fat.

A lack of vital nutrients can cause mental fatigue, low energy, and a decreased sex drive. The following 6 key nutrients will help you lose weight, maintain a healthy weight, and help you to maintain vital health.

1. Feel Full With Fiber

Even though the recommended daily intake of fiber is at least 25g, most people only eat about 15g of fiber per day. Fiber helps you feel fuller longer.

A higher fiber intake helps prevent heart disease, some types of cancer (such as cancer of the colon), constipation, and Type 2 diabetes.

Fruit, vegetables, whole grain cereals, and legumes are all good sources of fiber. Drink plenty of water to avoid feeling bloated and gassy as you increase your fiber intake.

2. Omega-3 Fatty Acids

Not all fats are the same. Some fats consumed in moderate amounts are actually healthy. A deficiency in omega-3 fatty acids can cause dry skin and depression, as well as increasing your risk of heart disease.

You can find omega-3 fatty acids in nuts, avocados, cold-water fish such as salmon, and egg whites. Omega-3 fatty acids can help you feel full longer, reducing the urge to snack. If these foods don't thrill you, add an omega-3 fatty acids supplement to your diet to increase your intake of this vital nutrient. For added benefit, add Omega 6 & 9 fatty acids too.

3. Folic Acid

Pregnant women aren't the only ones who need folic acid. Everyone needs at least 400 micrograms of folic acid per day. Whole grain products such as cereals and breads are usually fortified with folic acid. Folic acid protects you from colon cancer, and heart disease.

4. Calcium

You need 1,000 milligrams of calcium per day. Calcium makes bones strong. It can also help with weight loss, and it can help regulate blood pressure.

5. Vitamin D

Vitamin D helps with the absorption of calcium; it fights some abnormal cells by boosting your immune system. The daily recommended dose is 200mg although this is believed to be far too low and many practitioners are recommending 1000mg a day.

6. Iron

If you're suffering from low energy, you may have an iron-deficiency. Iron helps your red blood cells carry oxygen through the body. Take an iron supplement, and/or eat iron-rich foods such as spinach, seafood, beans, etc. Vitamin C will increase your iron absorption, as will taking it on an empty stomach.

A Healthy Lifestyle

A healthy lifestyle will improve your quality of life regardless of your age. Regular exercises, not smoking, drinking minimal amounts of alcohol, eating healthy, and reducing stress in your life are all essential to a healthy lifestyle.

Did you know that people, who are physically active for 30 minutes a day, control their weight, eat healthy foods, and refrain from smoking reduce their risk factors for most chronic diseases by up to 80%?

Low Impact Exercise

Physical activity is an essential part of a healthy lifestyle. Just 30 minutes a day will do it, and that can be broken into 10-minute intervals, if you insist.

The benefits of physical activity affect you from the inside out. Some health improvements occur gradually and so you may not notice them right away, while other changes you'll be aware of almost instantly, such as increased energy.

Small changes to your physical activity can make a significant difference in the way you look and feel.

Being physically active doesn't mean you have to participate in sports. Low impact exercises such as swimming or walking can give you all the benefits. If you have a dog, you can make walking the dog a family activity for physical exercise.

Here, are some of the health benefits that occur from making physical activity a part of your daily life.

- ☑ Helps maintain a healthy body weight
- ☑ Improves your mental state
- ☑ Helps control blood pressure
- ☑ Lowers risk of Type 2 diabetes
- ☑ Reduces stress
- ☑ Builds stronger bones and tones muscles
- ☑ Improves balance and posture
- ☑ Increases resistance to disease
- ☑ Improves cholesterol levels
- ☑ Improves the quality of sleep
- ☑ Reduces the chance of a heart attack
- ☑ Improves self-esteem and confidence
- ☑ Increases relaxation

☑ Increases energy
☑ Reduces feelings of anxiety/depression

Treat the Body Right

You need to give your body the same attention you would give to the functioning of your sports car. If you failed to put oil into your Ferrari, it would quickly grind to a halt. If you put the wrong kind of oil or gasoline into your Ferrari, it would also fail you.

If you left that car in the sun by the seaside, the surface would readily rust if it were not painted and otherwise covered with a special protectant. The other fluids – transmission fluid etc, need to be attended to, or the other aspects of the vehicle will fail too. Waxing the car will keep the paint from fading.

The driver of such a car would have to be appropriately attired to drive the car. It wouldn't be right for the Ferrari owner to be going to a gala performance in a t-shirt and jeans, *unless of course they lived in Seattle.*

So by the same token, it is necessary to treat your various body parts right. You need the right shoes to protect your feet from the environment or your activity. If you are going to be standing all day, jogging, mountain climbing, or walking on coral reefs, you need the right kind of shoes.

Similarly, one wouldn't ask a bare body to go out into the frozen weather of Edmonton, Alberta, Canada in mid winter. You have to wrap it with woolens, or other thermal maintaining fabrics. On the other hand, in the heat of Florida, one wears light cottons, so the body can breathe and function correctly.

CHAPTER 3

COMPLIMENTARY THERAPIES

East Meets West

For many years now, health care professionals in the western world have been looking at how those in eastern parts of the world take care of their patients, in hopes of delivering a better quality of health care here in the west.

There are many who have jumped aboard the "Alternative Care, Complementary Care, New Age" medicine bandwagon. Some in response to surveys that indicate that patients in western countries are dissatisfied with the quality, cost, and ineffectiveness of western (allopathic) medicine in addressing <u>certain</u> conditions.

Others have joined the alternative bandwagon, because their patients have come to their offices with bottles of formerly strange sounding items asking their doctor to incorporate this or that treatment into their current allopathic treatment regime. In some cases, they are simply asking if it will interfere with their current allopathic treatments.

Unfortunately, some practitioners have joined the movement for purely financial reasons. Still others have joined the movement because of a genuine belief that there are alternative treatments out there, which can honestly assist in the treatment of some conditions.

Many individuals, myself included, look at products and methodologies with a critical eye. In science, and I am speaking of basic science, we insist on a scientific research method being applied to all potential products our patients are going to use.

This method is quite simple. It dictates that anything that is to be believed must be proven by a controlled experiment. This means that depending on the specific study, you start with a large group of individuals who share similar characteristics pertaining to age, size; health status; etc.

Then one applies the product or method to be examined to one part of the group, while the other group receives a placebo (a fake). By studying the results, one can determine if there is a statistically significant difference between the two groups. If there is a significant positive difference, one can determine if there is any advantage to utilizing the new product or not. We will discuss scientific studies further in other chapters.

Many of us doctors who have looked at other methodologies and medications have done so because we have wanted to find a gentler way of dealing with disease. In some instances, these treatments do a better job of dealing with the human body than our current western, allopathic medicine does.

I will be the first to be a proponent for allopathic medicine in situations of an urgent nature; such as accidents, burns, heart attacks, overwhelming infections, strokes, fractures, major cancers, and the like.

Our western medicine has excelled in diagnosing the extent of these conditions and expeditiously treating them.

The aspect of medicine where we seem to be lacking in western medicine is in a variety of chronic diseases and in prevention of them in the first place. My personal observation of many of the eastern medical practices is that over the centuries they have excelled at addressing some of the problems of chronic disease.

This is not to say that Asia is the only place where gentler practices occur. In my studies, I have also observed very effective practices that have emanated from a variety of native peoples in North, Central and South America. I have also seen certain practices labeled alternative in Western Europe, just recently gaining recognition in mainstream Western–American medicine.

It is these practices that are incorporated into my methodology of treating patients, and preventing disease. Let me emphasize that my belief system is not fixed. Daily, I am introduced to new and exciting methodologies.

Ever since I began researching various medical practices, lecturing and writing about them, there is one thing that I have learned as a constant: nothing is constant and there is always something new that may have some application to some disease process for someone. Similarly, there may be something that we need to stop doing or throw out.

I have also learned that there are many substances and practices that can encourage the body to treat it. The human body is a marvelous machine. If you treat it right, it will perform beautifully.

Again, let us use the example of a sports car. If you tune the machine perfectly, it will hum and perform the way it was designed to do – specific speeds can be attained, the proper handling characteristics will be met, the proper temperature of the oil will be maintained, and the ambient climate for the inhabitant will be optimized.

If on the other hand, you use bad tires, the overall experience of driving in the vehicle will not be as pleasant as it could be.

One can readily see where this can be like the human body. Give it the wrong food/fuel, fail to change improper habits/oil, fail to use the correct clothing for the climate or activity/tires, and damage will occur to blood, organs, or muscles/bones/skin in the same way it does the sports car. Treat it right, and it will hum into old age without many of the problems some people have.

Staying with the sports car image, most of us are familiar with preventive maintenance. The same thing applies to the human body. If you utilize various methodologies and substances, you will be able to better fight off future problems such as diseases that you are exposed to in your daily life, various digestive problems, and problems with the musculoskeletal system.

Many of the herbs and teas used in Asia are designed to act in strengthening the immune system so that problems in the future can be eliminated or at the very least, brushed off by the immune system when the body is attacked.

I recall shopping for a car for my parents after they were involved in an accident. My dad was used to driving a small sized car, and so when I suggested a full sized "boat" as added protection to his driving techniques, he was completely against it.

When I read about one smaller sized car brand that had built in side protection, side air bags, a resilient coating on the doors, I encouraged my dad to purchase this vehicle, and he did so. Over several years, it was able to "brush off" many of my dad's driving indiscretions with walls, curbs, and the like; and one hopes in a more serious mishap that it would have protected the inhabitants of the car.

The designers of the car, built up its' "immune system" to help ward off potential problems much as we need to with the human body. For example, Astragalus, a root found in Asia, does a similar thing with the human body. We will discuss this type of substance in detail in later chapters.

Even when you take immaculate care of yourself, and you never do anything stupid in the way of extracurricular activities, accidents still happen and the body needs to be repaired. Fractures have to be set, burns have to be treated, and infections have to be attended to. This is where allopathic medicine comes to the forefront and excels in assisting individuals diminishing the accidents' effects.

There are also situations where a person chooses to have elective surgical procedures, that also require healing. Plastic surgical procedures, for example, can effectively treat vanity issues or acquired deformities.

I have found that in addition to the appropriate surgical, bacteriologic, and first aid measures used in western medicine to attend to these procedures, various methods and treatments commonly used in Asian medicine can allow the body to heal faster, more naturally and often with less discomfort.

The old adage taught to us in medical school still applies: **do no harm**. Combine this with my adage: **help the body to heal itself**.

When you allow that to happen, you will be surprised at how the body will rally to help itself. All it needs is a helping hand with proper direction. This book is designed to give you, the potential patient, exactly that – a helping hand with self directed suggestions, and advice on questions to ask your physician.

I will show you items that may be incorporated into your current treatment regime. This book will also direct you the reader to various techniques and treatment places throughout the world, in which various aspects discussed here, are practiced.

As this book is being written, I am sure there are new places that are being opened that will have innovative ways of treating and preventing disease. In just one book, I cannot hope to cover all aspects of the healing arts, and all of the places where the reader could potentially receive these types of treatments, but it is my goal to provide you with the knowledge to get started, and to sort out the wheat from the shaft. In future books, I will address other issues.

As the body ages, it changes. This simple fact means you have to change what you do to and for your body. Exercise that was appropriate when we were 18 is usually not appropriate for the average 50 year old.

Even if we keep our body well tuned, there are changes that will occur, and it is important that you adjust to those changes, in order to avoid damaging various body systems and so that you can prevent further degeneration, as much as possible.

Aromatherapy

Aromatherapy is designed to help balance and harmonize the human mind, body and spirit with the controlled use of pure essential oils in such a way as to restore and maintain good health and a feeling of well-being.

Essential oils are derived from plants and contain an energy and life force with it's own medicinal properties. Many of these oils are antiseptic, antifungal and antibacterial.

They generally have no side effects, and help alleviate various stress related conditions, musculoskeletal conditions, and some psychological conditions.

Aromatherapy is the practice of using the natural oils, which are extracted from flowers, roots, stems, bark, leaves, or other parts of a plant, and is said to improve psychological and physical well-being.

The inhaled aroma from the essential oils is said to stimulate your brain function. Essential oils can also be absorbed through your skin, traveling through your blood stream, and providing healing qualities to the whole body.

Aromatherapy was slow to catch on but as more, and more people experience its benefits its popularity has begun to grow. Aromatherapy can be used to soothe the mind, as a mood enhancement to improve cognitive function, aid in sleep, and for pain relief.

There are a many essential oils available. Each of the oils has their own healing properties. Full dictionaries are available to guide the person wanting to use this health technique.

Homeopathy

Homeopathy is a two hundred year old system of complementary medicine. It originated in Germany as a gentle system of treatment with presumably no major side effects.

Its proponents profess that it addresses the entire person, the physical and emotional aspects of the person including the signs and symptoms that the person is presenting with.

Homeopathic medicines are mostly made from plants or minerals and are given in extremely diluted doses to avoid side effects. The treatment is based on the theory that 'symptoms are expressions of a disharmony within the whole person.'

The remedies are prescribed to produce minute symptoms matching those of the disease. This theoretically brings about the neutralization of the symptom thereby balancing the individual's energy system.

The term homeopathy comes from the Greek words homeo, meaning similar, and pathos, meaning suffering or disease. Homeopathy seeks to stimulate the body's ability to heal itself by giving tiny doses of a highly diluted substance. German physician Samuel Christian Hahnemann developed this therapy at the end of the 18th century. Hahnemann expressed two key principles:

The principle of similars (or "like cures like") states that a substance that produces similar symptoms in healthy people can cure a disease. This idea can be traced back to Hippocrates.

Hahnemann further developed the idea, after he repeatedly ingested cinchona bark, a popular treatment for malaria, and found that he developed symptoms of the disease. Hahnemann theorized that if a substance could cause disease symptoms in a healthy person, small amounts could potentially cure a sick person who had similar symptoms.

The homeopathic principle of dilutions or "law of minimum dose" says that the lower the dose of the medication, the greater its effectiveness. In homeopathy, substances are diluted in a stepwise method, and then shaken vigorously between each dilution. This process, referred to as "potentization," is believed to transmit some form of information or energy from the original substance to the final diluted remedy.

Most homeopathic remedies are so dilute that no molecules of the substance remain. However, homeopathy believes that the substance has left its essence, which will stimulate the body to heal itself. This theory is called "the memory of water."

Regulation of Homeopathic Remedies

Homeopathic remedies are prepared according to the guidelines of the Homeopathic Pharmacopeia of the United States (HPUS), which was written into law in the Federal Food, Drug, and Cosmetic Act in 1938. Homeopathic remedies are regulated in the same manner as over-the-counter drugs.

However, because homeopathic products contain little or no active ingredients, they do not have to undergo the same safety testing as prescription allopathic and new over the counter (OTC) drugs.

The U.S. Food and Drug Administration require that homeopathic remedies meet certain legal standards for strength, purity, and packaging. The labels on the remedies must include at least one major indication. For example, it must list at least one medical problem the remedy is used to treat.

It must also contain a list of ingredients, the dilution, and safety instructions. In addition, if a homeopathic remedy claims to treat a serious disease such as cancer, it needs to be sold by prescription. Only products for self-limiting conditions, such as headaches or colds, can be sold without a prescription.

Homeopathic Research

Homeopathy is difficult to study using current scientific methods because it is impossible to measure highly diluted substances. This makes it hard to create and/or replicate studies.

In addition, homeopathic treatments are highly individualized, which means the prescribing standard is inconsistent. There are hundreds of different homeopathic remedies, which can be prescribed in a variety of different dilutions to treat thousands of symptoms.

On the other hand, many aspects of the interactions between the homeopathic practitioner and his/her patients may be quite beneficial and can be studied more easily.

Homeopathy is a controversial area of alternative medicine, because a number of its key concepts are not consistent with established laws of science, particularly chemistry and physics.

Critics believe it is unlikely that a remedy containing such a tiny amount of any active ingredient can have any biological effect—beneficial or otherwise. Critics maintain that continuing the scientific study of homeopathy is not worthwhile.

Still others point to observational evidence that homeopathy does work, and they feel that it should not be discounted, or rejected just because science has not been able to explain it.

Homeopathic Side Effects and Risks

While risks and side effects associated with homeopathic remedies have not had adequate research, there are some general points regarding homeopathic treatment safety.

- Homeopathic remedies in high dilution, taken under the supervision of trained professionals, are considered generally safe, and unlikely to cause any serious adverse reactions.

- Liquid homeopathic remedies may contain alcohol. The FDA allows higher levels of alcohol in these remedies than it allows in conventional drugs. However, no adverse effects from alcohol levels have been reported to the FDA.

- Homeopathic practitioners feel some patients may experience a temporary worsening of their symptoms after taking a homeopathic prescription. Researchers have not been able to confirm this in clinical studies. However, homeopathic research is scarce.

While it does not appear that homeopathic remedies interfere with conventional drugs, if you are considering using homeopathic remedies, you should always talk to your allopathic physician first.

Reiki

Reiki is a Japanese method of healing which has been in existence for many centuries. Reiki in Japanese means "universal life energy" and refers to the energy that flows through all living beings.

The word Reiki is made of two Japanese words – Rei, which means "God's Wisdom or the Higher Power" and Ki, which is "life force energy". Reiki is "spiritually guided life force energy."

A typical Reiki treatment involves the practitioner allowing energy to flow through them to the patient by calling on a higher power, much like the treatments that Native healers use in Canada and the USA. A treatment is said to feel like a "wonderful glowing radiance that flows through and around you".

Reiki claims to treat the whole person including mind, body, and spirit, as well as emotions creating many beneficial effects that include relaxation and feelings of peace, security, and wellbeing. Many have reported miraculous results.

It is said to make all cells of the body come into balance, stabilizing energy and releasing stress. There is deep relaxation with Reiki treatment. It is said that the whole body is treated so that energy can go to the source of the imbalance not just to the manifest symptoms.

Reiki is a simple, natural, and safe method of spiritual healing, and self-improvement that everyone should be able use. It claims to be effective in helping virtually every known illness. This type of claim always makes one suspect, especially when there are no scientifically supported studies. Since it appears not to do any harm, it should be able to be used with other medical or therapeutic techniques to promote recovery without any problems.

While Reiki is spiritual in nature, it is not a religion. It has no dogma, and there is no particular religion you must believe in, in order to learn or use Reiki. Because Reiki is said to come from God, many people find that using Reiki puts them more in touch with the experience of their religion, rather than only having an intellectual concept of it.

If one reads work by Dr. Mikao Usui, the founder of Reiki, one will quickly see that his message is one that contains some universally accepted truths that we all should follow. Many religious and health leaders recommended that everyone should practice certain simple ethical ideals to promote peace and harmony.

Reiki does so by stating that in order for the Reiki healing energies to have lasting results, the client must accept responsibility for his/her healing and take an active part in it.

Therefore, the Usui system of Reiki also includes an active commitment to improving oneself. The ideals are both guidelines for living a gracious life, and virtues worthy of practice for their inherent value.

Shiatsu

'Shi' means 'finger' and 'Atsu' means 'pressure'; Shiatsu literally means 'finger pressure', although in the actual practice of Shiatsu, almost every part of a practitioner's body is used to give this technique of energy massage to the receiver.

While its historical roots can be traced to China, it evolved into a distinct art in Japan over hundreds of years. Originally based on the principals of traditional Chinese medicine, it is now integrated with

Western philosophy. Unlike most Western forms of bodywork massage, Shiatsu is usually performed on a mat on the floor like Ayurveda.

The techniques used include yoga like stretches, soft tissue massage and the use of acupressure along the meridian energy channels that are classic in Chinese medicine. It is a therapy, which can be adapted to a variety of conditions.

It is said that Shiatsu balances the body's energy flow activating the person's natural healing mechanisms. It apparently helps improve circulation, releases muscle tension and aids all around flexibility of the individual.

Ayurveda

Ayurveda is a scientific knowledge from India rooted in over five thousand years of time-honored traditions and practices.

Ayurveda means "the science of life" in Sanskrit, culled from the Atharva Veda, the fourth and last of the sacred Hindu texts called the Rig Veda. Over the centuries, Ayurveda has influenced many western modalities of healing such as homeopathy, aromatherapy, psychiatry, meditation, & nutrition.

Ayurveda recognizes that every individual has a unique psycho-physiological make-up, with his or her own basic constitution from conception on. It promotes customized self-healing, with the assistance of a trained practitioner.

As with many practitioners who attempt to meld the lines between western and eastern medicine, those who practice Ayurveda show the interrelatedness of body-mind-spirit in promoting overall good health in a person. To be practiced properly, Ayurveda needs the guidance of a trained practitioner.

Ayurveda is based upon three constitutional types or doshas: vata, pita, and kapha. These constituents balance out the person, by bestowing a state of good health, happiness, and a sense of well-being.

It is said that instead of dealing with pathogens (organisms that contribute to disease) and trying to destroy them, Ayurveda works on strengthening the immune system; much the same theory as other systems that attempt to assist the body in trying to heal itself.

In Ayurveda, food is thought to be very important, because food and its components make up the body's cells and tissues. As I have said many times, we are what we eat.

Ayurveda also address lifestyle practices that may drain and weaken a person's vitality. Ayurveda feels that the stress in our modern lives is harmful to the body because it does not give the body time to balance with quiet time, and down time. As with many eastern approaches to health, rest and meditation are part of the treatment.

As with many philosophies, Ayurveda teaches that you must live each day consciously and with a positive attitude. It says that you can do this by unlocking the life force called prana (similarly called qi in Chinese).

- ☑ It is up to the individual to consciously want to make positive decisions that impact a quality of life that has vibrant, healing energy

- ☑ A person's immune system becomes powerful from a balanced body-mind-spirit that then radiates outer vitality and good health.

Ayurvedic Vocabulary

Every medical field has its' own vocabulary. Ayurveda has an ancient and descriptive vocabulary that is needed to understand the intricacies of the practice.

Abhyanga	A term used to describe an Ayurvedic oil massage practiced by two medics who massage to let go the warm oil into the tissues of the entire body. This helps to loosen and help the removal of accumulated toxins and the Doshas (Vata, Pitta, and Kapha) from the body.
Agni	The form of fire and heat that is the basis of the digestive system and the process of release of energy. The term includes the body heat, body temperature, sight, the digestive fire; its function is transformation, absorption, elimination and discrimination is Agni.
Ama	It is the toxins that enter the blood stream and are circulated in the whole body. Toxins or ama are produced in the body by the raw, undigested food products that become fetid. Toxins are vital for prana (vital life energy), ojas (immunity), and tejas (cell metabolic energy).
Apa	The element water.
Apana	One of the five types of Vata, which goes downward and is responsible for expulsion of feces, flatus, urine, menstrual blood etc.
Asana	Yoga posture – the third limb of Yoga.

Ayurveda	Constituted of two words, Ayur meaning life and Veda meaning knowledge, ayurveda means the knowledge of life. Another accurate translation of ayurveda is the knowledge of longevity.
Atharva veda	The Atharva Veda compound of an ancient Rishi, and (meaning "knowledge") is a sacred text of Hinduism, and one of the four Vedas, often called the "fourth Veda.
Bala	This is a Sanskrit word which means strength.
Chakra	These are the energy centers in the body that are related to the nerve plexus center, which govern the body functions. Chakra meaning 'the wanderer' is believed to have spent many years between the wild animals in dense jungles, which enabled him to coin his experiences in the book considered as the bible of Ayurveda and called the Chakra Samhita.
Dhatu	It is the basic structural and nutritional body factor that supports, or nourishes the seven body tissues. These seven tissues of our body include the rasa, rakta, mamsa, meda, asthi, majja, and shukra.

Decoction	A method of extraction by boiling of dissolved chemicals, or herbal or plant material, which may include stems, roots, bark and rhizomes.
Dinacharya	Rejuvenation of the mind; daily practices.
Doshas	Three main forces which govern the body (Väta, Pitta and Kapha) literally means faulty or to cause harm, although they only do so when they are functioning abnormally.
Emesis	An act or instance of vomiting (a form of purgation)
Jala	Water, fluid.
Karma	Action; work; a complex concept, the word originally denoted a religious act or rite and gradually assumed other shades of meaning, as in, action, work, past actions as producing good or evil results; the accumulated effect of deeds in lives, past and present.
Katu	Pungent taste or flavor.
Gandharva	Celestial musicians. Heavenly singers.
Ghee	It is the clarified butter made by heating unsalted butter. The ghee may be stored without refrigeration and can be used for most of the preparations that need oil or butter as the basic ingredient.

Guna	All material entities including the mind are the composites of the three gunas, namely the sattva, rajjas and tamas.
Maha Bhutas	Yoga and Pancha The five senses have five dimensions in the universe.
Marma	These are the nerve crossings where nerves come to the fascia and relate to the vital human body organs. Marmas are the 365 vital energy points in the body of which 108 are of great importance in Ayurveda.
Nadi	Pulse, any tubular organ such as vein or artery.
Ojas	Vigor, strength and vitality that is the essence of all tissues (dhatus). It means the life sap or the essence of the immune system and spiritual energy. Ojas is a protoplasmic substance called the albumin and globulin that is formed during the biosynthesis of bodily tissues and strengthens the tissues.
Panchakarma	According to ayurveda this refers to the five cleansing therapies i.e. vaman, virechan, basti, nasya and rakta moksha. In literal terms, these internal purifications refer to vomiting, purgation, decoction enema, oily enema, and nasal medications

Pitta	It is one of the three Doshas i.e. the bile humor, entire hormones, enzymes, coenzymes and agencies responsible for the physiochemical processes of the body.
Pragnyaparadha	A mistake in the intellect and consciousness.
Prakriti	Unconscious, inherent relationship between self and matter. In other words it means one's life consumption.
Pranayama	It is a breathing exercise for purifying the blood and vitalizing the inner organs. The three aspects of this exercise are inhalation, retention, and exhalation with the aim of increasing the span of each aspect and more controlled.
Purification	Attain proper balance of vatha, pitha and kapha based on the panchkarma and swethakarma treatments.
Purgation	The purification or cleansing of someone or something
Rajas	The law of nature that maintains life. It is one of the three gunas characterized by action, energy, passion, and stimulation that lead to the life of sensual enjoyment, pleasure and pain, efforts and restlessness.

Quantum	
	Energetic frequencies used to balance the three Dosha and can help you identify the links to some of the impacts of imbalanced Doshas.
Rasas	Moisture, humidity
Rasayana	Rejuvenation
Rejuvenation	Helps to promote and preserve health and longevity.
Rishi	The composers of Vedic hymns. However, according to post-Vedic tradition, the rishi is a "seer" to whom the Vedas were "originally revealed" through states of higher consciousness.
Satva	Purity – First of the three gunas, it is the purest aspect and the sentient principle characterized by purity, luminosity, lightness, harmony and the production of pleasure.
Seer	By divine will and through the realization of the rishis (seers), Ayurveda was disseminated as a healing practice and a guide for living in harmony with the spirit of nature.
Surya Namaskara	The first sun salutation – five rounds for a start in a practice of Ashtanga Yoga. Its nine movements are shown here in pictures and text.
Tamas	Darkness, inertia, heaviness and the materialistic attitude.
Upaveda	Applied knowledge.

Vata	One of the three humors, the force that keeps pitta, kapha, all the seven dhatus and the malas in motion.
Vedic	Have or relating to the Veda or Vedas. The language of the Vedas, an early form of Sanskrit.
Vedas	Knowledge. Vedas are the oldest source of universal knowledge, which bloomed in the Indian culture centuries ago by rishis and holy saints. The four Vedas namely, Rig-Veda, Yajur Veda, Athrva Veda and Sam Veda have answers to mostly all questions relating to life and living.
Yoga	Derived from Sanskrit word "yug" which means to unite, to combine or to integrate.
Yogic	A Hindu discipline aimed at training the consciousness for a state of perfect spiritual insight and tranquility.

What the Bible Says About Healthy Living

In many religious traditions, there are pronouncements, and rules about what one should and should not eat and drink. Many of these pronouncements and rules are based upon the fact that, <u>at the time they were written</u>, one could get extremely ill from eating certain foods. No refrigeration existed, and the cradle of civilizations had warm climates.

The Jewish & Moslem faiths forbade pork, undoubtedly for that very reason. The Christians forbade sex with anyone other than ones wife- undoubtedly to stem the ever-present sexually transmitted diseases.

In the Christian Bible, there were many other pronouncements of a health related nature:

- ✓ In Corinthian's 6: 19, 20 – Our bodies belong to God; therefore, they are holy and should be treated as such.
- ✓ In Corinthian's 3:16, 17 – It says, we can defile the temples of our bodies by unhealthful practices including what we eat and drink.
- ✓ In John 2:3 – Communicates to us that we need to have healthy bodies and clear minds.
- ✓ In Genesis 1:29 – The original diet God gave human beings included fruits, nuts, and grains. 3:17 vegetables were added later.
- ✓ In Revelation 21:27 – Heaven will not contain anything that defiles or corrupts. This would certainly include recreational drugs, tobacco, and other unhealthful practices.
- ✓ In Corinthian 10:31 – Whatever we do, we are to do everything in a way that will glorify God and that includes what we eat or drink.

Meditation

Nature has a truly healing elixir. Just by looking out my east-facing window to drink in the morning sky awash in orange and pink against the canvas of an emerging dawn, I am invigorated -- no matter what the outside temperature may be. It gives me energy to greet and offer thanks for a new day ahead. And by intuitively doing this, it offers a soulful salutation and meditation to Mother Nature.

When I share this simple story in classes, students immediately identify with similar experiences that bring them joy from deep within—be they hiking and enjoying scenic views, or walking barefoot on a smooth, sandy beach. These are all types of meditation. Put simply, meditation is being transported to an inner space where mind, body, and spirit are comfortably at ease with one another. Nature's meditation, like music meditation, is spontaneous in bringing serenity to anyone who is receptive and open to inner quiet.

We only need go with the flow of the moment, by allowing ourselves to be transported to other realms of inner harmony—and in doing so; we release debilitating stress from our lives.

Meditation has been practiced in its many forms for centuries -- from hilltops in Tibet to monasteries in the Middle Ages in Europe. Jump forward a few centuries, and one will find many cultures that use one form or another of meditation in the 21st century. In the 1970's the Hippie culture embraced meditation in various forms. Some of the more scientific individuals of the New Age tested various forms of this 'meditation' and found that they could prove scientifically that there was medical/physiological benefits from meditation. It became all the rage in universities and hospitals. Transcendental Meditation (TM) became a major tool for Death & Dying counselors, Recreational Therapists, Cancer wards and psychologists in general. Studies of this, and other techniques, showed that regular periods of meditation improved not only the well being of the individual, but the blood pressure, alpha waves in the brain, etc. Meditation encompasses many techniques and theories of why it works.

A garden "can act as a healing place, where we can substitute soothing images for disturbing ones," Julie Messervy in *The Inward Garden* (1995), claims that gardening is a form of happy, healthy nature meditation that re-balances body-mind-spirit.
Another passionate gardener and designer who regularly appears on TV, Fran Sorin, writes in *Digging Deep: Unearthing Your Creative Roots Through Gardening* (2004), "Our creative roots make up the very fiber of who we are as individuals, and by unearthing our creative nature, we, at the same time, unearth our authentic selves. ... At the end of the day, the reason we create is not for the finished product, but to get to the best parts of ourselves."

What we do with love, sincerity, and intensity (or passion) also necessitates digging deep inwardly to achieve the most satisfying results. Sorin's and Messervy's garden metaphors drive home this point vividly.

Welcoming Nature's beauty into our lives can take other forms that are meditative, healing, and fulfilling, as well. Have you noticed how serene a quilter's living room feels? How tranquil a potter's studio is? And how earthy it smells? The uplifting aromas of freshly baked bread and chocolate chip cookies as they waft through your house? Taking the time to enjoy a cup of freshly brewed tea, while being reinvigorated, with subtle aromas that tantalize the nostrils and heighten the senses?

We can be as creatively meditative as we want to be, in whatever mode we enjoy—gardening, cooking, cleaning, reading, and running—in order to feel totally happy, at peace, secure, and fulfilled with our lives. This is simply the secret of inviting meditation into your daily activities, if only for a few moments daily – to be cleansed and purified by staying in the heart, and engaging in activities that rebalance us with new energy.

How to Meditate At Home, in the Office, etc.

Meditation is very easy for anyone who wants to rebalance the mind, body, and spirit. It will invite peaceful energy into your consciousness. Although those who have learned meditation well can meditate anywhere (I remember well, noting a local man meditating in the middle of a busy bus station in India), when you begin to learn to meditate, it is best to start in a quiet, peaceful place.

1. Unplug your home/office phone and turn off your cell phone.

2. Create an area that is clear of stuff, clean, and inviting. It can be in a corner somewhere in your house, by your bed, and even a space on your desk.

3. Create an ambiance, if you like, by having a beautiful picture, incense, flowers, etc. in the meditation area. Some techniques have you concentrate on a picture or other object.

4. Sit up straight, and in a comfortable position.

5. Loosen your clothing—unbutton, unbuckle; and kick off your shoes.

6. Start by loosening your neck and shoulder muscles. Do this by first turning your head clock-wise, and then counter-clockwise a few times.

7. You will feel the tension slowly dissipating.

8. Close your eyes

9. Rest your hands in your lap, so they are not distracting you.

10. Then, consciously breathe in deep and slow. The key to a breathing meditation is to consciously breathe deeply and to expel all your old energy.

11. Begin by inhaling – count—one, two—for peaceful energy to enter into your body. Hold for the count of three, four. You will feel this new energy expanding into every pore of your being. Now gently exhale—five, six—as you release restless energy back to the universe. Continue repeating, until you feel the new waves of energy purifying your whole being. You will then be inhaling, and exhaling peaceful energy.

12. Now begin thinking a word. As Herbert Benson MD (Harvard Press) suggests in his book, it can be as simple as the word "one". If you are a Buddist Monk, Hindu Yogi, TM Meditator, Christian Monk or other, your teacher will give you a special word, or mantra. These are word sounds that have been used for centuries to help people achieve a deep meditative state. But without these traditions, you can use the word "one", "God", "love", "Christ", etc, etc. The key is to just think the word repetitively, over and over in your mind. When other thoughts enter your mind, sweep them out and return to thinking the special word. An experienced meditator will be able to stop at a designated 15 or 20 minutes (sufficient time for the mind to gain a good rest), but for newcomers and anyone who is very tired, set a quiet alarm or get someone to arouse you gently. Then be sure to include quiet time after each session, to better assimilate your experiences, before re-entering into the hustle and bustle of life.

If you find yourself hungry before you begin to meditate, eat a piece of fruit and/or drink water but do not eat a full meal before meditating.

Applications of Meditation Techniques

You can use meditation to refresh sagging spirits, or whenever you feel the need for some new energy to continue with the day's activities.

3 O'clock Meditation

Another variation is the "3'o clock Meditation." Instead of reaching for calorie filled snacks that provide momentary gratification and lasting effect, enjoy instead increased energy, minus the calories by:

Closing your eyes momentarily. Breathing in deeply, consciously, feel this expansive surge of pure powerful energy, revitalizing your body-mind consciousness and blessing your entire being. Breathe in the renewed vigor as your toes tingle, and warm waves of love and appreciation begins to gently stir in your heart.

Guidelines to Knowing Your Mediation is Working

Meditation is the normal birthright of every person. Learning to meditate is like getting re-acquainted with an old friend again; it's easy to reconnect. Your inner pilot is your best guide —so go with your intuitive responses, and learn to listen from within to your innermost self, to your own soul's light. Some guidelines that meditation is working are:

✓ When you feel a deep sense of well-being, from the very depths of your heart especially right after a meditation.

✓ When your mind is at peace, and not contradicting nor dictating your heartfelt feelings welling up from within.

✓ When you relax, and entrust your inner pilot to instinctively guide you to breathe deeply, have faith in your meditation taking you on to new adventures, and letting go of expectations of how meditation ought to proceed.

✓ If you meditate correctly, you will feel spontaneous inner joy and peace within and without.

✓ If you find yourself feeling mental tension or a disturbance, then the type of meditation you are doing is not right for you-try a different technique.

✓ When you have a good meditation, you will have a good feeling for the world. You will see the world in a loving way in spite of all the imperfections you are aware of.

Don't be upset if you are unable to meditate well in the beginning. Even in the outer life, God alone knows how many years one must practice in order to become adept at something.

Three Meditation Questions:

✓ **How long should I meditate?** Begin with 15 to 20 minutes at a time. The key is to focus on your meditation without being distracted by thoughts and anxieties, just go back to your special word.

✓ **When should I meditate?** Anytime is ok but generally from a medical point of view you should meditate 2 times a day. As morning shows the beginning of a new day, do a morning meditation. It can pave the way for a brand new day ahead with new aspirations to live life purposefully and with a deep sense of satisfaction. Before lunch, and at the end of the workday or around sunset, are also excellent times as you can empty your consciousness of the day, along with the accumulated emotional baggage of the day.

✓ **How often should I meditate?** Try to meditate two times a day, but if possible, as often as the inner you beckons— In other words, whenever you feel an intuitive tune-up to rebalance your life by becoming more calm and focused.

Is Meditation Practical?

If you are practical in your inner life, by praying, and meditating, then you will increase your inner awareness. When you have inner awareness, you have free access to infinite truth and everlasting joy. You are then able to control your outer life.

You always grow from within, not from without. It is from the seed under the ground that a plant grows, not vice versa. The inner life constantly carries the message of truth and God. The inner truth is the seed.

It doesn't matter how many hours you do anything in the outer world, but if you first meditate then act and speak afterwards, your actions will be enriched by your meditation.

Rejuvenation

In the context of health, rejuvenation is considered a rebirth of the body to perfect health.

    ✓ Rejuvenation in Ayurveda is called Rasayana.

    ✓ Rejuvenation from the point of view of the American Indian is a rebirth of spirit and body by removing evil spirits.

    ✓ Rejuvenation in Western medicine during the middle ages was achieved by bloodletting and removing the evil humors that were thought to create disease.

    ✓ In Irian Jaya, certain of the cannibalistic tribes believe that eating the bodies of stronger humans can rejuvenate them. In reality, I observed a number of them ending up with various diseases that the other Tribesmen had and dying in the process!

Even in the 21st-century's allopathic Western medicine, there is an underlying belief that rejuvenation of various body systems can be attained by removal of "offending substances".

This can be seen when we perform various types of chemotherapeutics, bone marrow transplants, ABO incompatibility transfusions, etc. In other words, medical science hasn't really changed much over the centuries and is not particularly different in many parts of the world when you get to the core of our beliefs.

Rejuvenation has become a hugely popular buzzword in Western Europe and throughout North America. One sees relatively healthy young people going to centers where they are given a variety of treatments to become rejuvenated. This can take the form of diet, massage, meditation, detoxification, purgation, etc.

Some of these techniques can certainly be justified in being appropriate treatment for somebody who has been on any dietary or drug binge. Certainly western doctors would agree that in detoxifying a chronic alcoholic, that certain measures, including psychological and physical counseling would be appropriate in being able to rejuvenate the individual.

When one carefully looks at all of these new rejuvenation processes, one sees a common thread. Basically, one is trying to harmonize the functions of the body by modulating the neuroendocrine immune function.

In other words, this means that one is trying to strengthen the individuals' general resistance to disease by stimulating the immune system of the body. By doing so, the individual will certainly feel much more alive and invigorated.

If one has a chronic disease, and this can be modulated, there is a decent chance that this rejuvenation will make one feel better. If one is otherwise generally healthy, recharging the system through a rejuvenation process, one will feel even healthier

We will discuss the role of stress, and emotions throughout this book. It is a well-known fact that stress and emotions play a role in immunological dysfunction.

It is also known that stress has an intimate role in the pathogenesis of many diseases. Consequently, if one is to rejuvenate the body by increasing the immuno competence of that body, it makes sense that the tissues could then sustain the effects of external and internal stress more easily.

CHAPTER 4

THE PROCESS OF AGING

Aging is a natural process that starts the day we are born. Now that I have stated the obvious, let me reiterate it in a different way.

The human body changes with age. It degenerates; falls apart, diminishes in strength, and looses elasticity. In other words, we get old.

The March of Time

The unrelenting march of time applies to every organ system of the body. From the day we are born, the system starts and we begin to age.

✓ Our muscles get weaker, and we are not able to stretch as well because the connective tissue tightens up.

✓ Our vision gets weaker and begins to blur due to degeneration in parts of the eye.

✓ Our joints degenerate not allowing the stability we were once accustomed to, and we feel pain when we try to carry out what had once been normal activity.

✓ Our digestion is not as efficient as before. Certain foods no longer agree with the body, creating discomforts, and depositing their residues in places we would prefer they would not.

✓ Our body hair begins to fall out in some places while we tend to gain it in other places.

✓ Our body fat redistributes itself. We appear more like plump pears perched upon overly sturdy piano legs rather than graceful birds ready to take flight.

✔ Our skin demonstrates the effects of many years of exposure to ultraviolet light, and other environmental modifiers in either very colorful palates, or very serious growths.

✔ Our skeletal structure loses its minerals and consequently becomes weaker and prone to fractures that are difficult to repair.

✔ Our ligaments that support that skeletal system give way, allowing further injury to the already weakened joints.

✔ Our body shows the effects of environmental exposures that create growths in parts of the body. These tumors can sometimes quickly put an end to an otherwise productive life.

✔ The human brain also ages by losing its structure on a daily basis. This, along with other unknown factors can lead to conditions that can allow the rest of the body to survive, while at the same time, totally devastating the thinking process of the brain with conditions such as Alzheimer's.

✔ Our dietary habits and indiscretions can change our physical appearance, and cause some of our organs to function improperly. Consequently this makes other systems fail, which is commonly seen in diabetes and coronary heart disease.

Let's face it – God created a formidable machine, but failed to give us ALL the tools necessary to keep that engine in perfect running order.

Sometimes we are given the education and wisdom to know how to keep that engine in prime condition so that it will not age as rapidly, but we consciously or unconsciously choose not to follow the suggestions.

In this book, I will discuss potential ways to help decrease the inevitable changes that occur with aging. It is your choice as to whether or not you follow them. Over and over I've told patient's what they can do to slow the aging process. Whether they take that advice or not isn't totally different question.

Obviously, there are also other reasons that people do not choose to follow recommendations of their health care professionals. Many underlying psychological and psychiatric aspects of the human mind surface, or lie dormant in ways that affect the persons' behavior toward medical issues.

This is why there is a medical specialty of psychiatry, and why there are medical physicians on staff at mental institutes. Mental changes that occur in the ageing individual encompass a delicate balance between perceived and real and the physical/chemical ability of the human brain to cope with those changes.

On many occasions during my career I have had the opportunity to work as a ship's physician. I have had the opportunity to observe a variety of ways in which a selected aging population addresses some of the physiological changes that the process throws at them. Some do it gracefully while others fight it in less than practical or healthy ways.

- Silver hair vs. bleached blondes

- Fish face vs. plastic surgery

- The 400+ pounders eating in excess, using their scooters to access every buffet, and growing in size by the day vs. the eater with hardly enough food on their plate to feed a sparrow.

- The exercise nuts vs. those that can be found in smoke filled rooms exercising one arm as they puff away.

- The free booze that lets the passenger stay drunk all day as a way of psychologically dealing with the inevitable death that will come, vs. the psychological games that people play, and the petty, childlike things that some do (stealing quiz points in trivia games) to make themselves feel important.

When the Body Ages

When the body ages, there are a number of significant changes that occur in various body systems. Many older individuals find themselves on a number of medications for various ailments. This is often referred to as "polypharmacy".

There can be some serious consequences from taking too many drugs, not taking the appropriate drugs, or taking the wrong drugs together, in the ageing body. The main problems with this polypharmacy are:

1. Adverse (abnormal) drug reactions to the drugs themselves Interactions between two drugs that are being taken in the same body.

2. Not taking the drugs at the right time or with the right food or liquid, which tends to be a greater problem when the drug regimens get more complicated.

3. Medication errors – taking too many of one medication and not enough of another.

4. Potential for physiological reactions in the aging body.

This latter issue, a potential for physiological reactions in the ageing body, is a real concern for western allopathic medications, homeopathic, naturopathic, and herbal based remedies alike.

There are age related factors that can change the metabolism of everything from allopathic drugs to vitamins, and everything in-between.

These changes in the body, and how the body reacts require that there be modifications to the selection, timing and dosing of the drug/vitamin/herbal material, which we will refer to generically as 'drug'. A knowledgeable allopathic physician and/or pharmacist may help prevent some of these potential problems.

Changes to Our Senses

We all know that the body changes with age. So far, in this chapter, we've covered some of the aspects of aging, and we will discuss it throughout the book in many forms.

Right now we are going to look at the changes that occur in smelling, tasting, hearing, and our eyesight as well as how the metabolism of various drugs that are taken can affect us when we are older.

The Sense of Smell/Taste

As any general practitioner can attest to, the sense of smell declines with aging. Unfortunately a number of the patient's in his waiting room will also attest to the fact that certain individuals have lost their sense of smell (or just don't like taking baths). The olfactory nerve endings in the nasal cavity become less efficient. Certain medical conditions will also decrease the sense of smell such as Alzheimer's, hypothyroidism, dementia, snorting cocaine, and even certain vitamin deficiencies, which we cover under diet.

As we get older, we lose the number of taste sensors and their functionality decreases. People who have been smokers or have folic acid deficiency will also tend to lose their sense of taste.

Aging Vision

As you get older, your eyes will have an increased sensitivity to glare, and you will experience a reduction in peripheral vision. Wearing glasses that reduce glare can sometimes help.

The risk of cataracts also increases with age. This is the result of irreversible changes in the proteins of the lens of the eye. This is one area in which antioxidants have been shown to reduce the damage to the proteins in the lens by neutralizing the free radicals. Although controlled studies have not been done, antioxidant supplements are most likely a prudent way of decreasing potential damage to the eyes.

As we age, it takes us longer to focus on an object. This is due to the increasing ocular muscle twitches and the time between each twitch slowing down our rate of focus.

Warning Signs of Age-related Vision Loss

While gradual vision loss may be an inevitable part of aging, you can slow down the damage to your vision, and in some cases even reverse it with proper care.

As you age you are more susceptible to conditions of the eye that can lead to permanent blindness, which is why it is important to have your eyes checked regularly, and see your ophthalmologist if you have any of the warning signs.

Trouble Reading or Doing Fine Work

Around the age of 40, presbyopia affects most people. It is why most of us begin to need reading glasses or bifocals. When the muscles get weak or the lens of the eye becomes stiff, your ability to read or do close up work diminishes, and you require reading glasses.

However, this isn't the only reason you may lose your ability to see fine details. The center of your retina, called the macula, is the area of the eye, which processes fine details. Some serious eye conditions, such as age related macular degeneration (AMD) and diabetic retinopathy, could also affect the macula of your eye. Initially these conditions often share similar symptoms to presbyopia, but quite quickly they can progress to permanent vision loss or blindness.

Seeing Stars or Shadows

A small amount of floaters can develop over the years, and they are considered normal and harmless. However, a sudden flood of floaters, stars, or a large shadow or veil over a portion of your vision, may indicate you have a tear in your retina or retinal detachment.

Retinal detachments are a medical emergency. Seek treatment right away. The delay of treatment by just a few hours can result in permanent vision loss.

Your Prescription Changes Frequently

It is normal for your vision to decline gradually as you age. However, the need for frequent changes in your prescription, or rapidly worsening vision, can be a sign of many eye conditions. It may be as simple as cataracts, or it may be something far more serious, such as diabetic retinopathy.

With diabetic retinopathy, the onset of vision loss is often the first symptom that a person has to alert them that they suffer from diabetes. This is just one of many dangerous health conditions that <u>rapid</u> changes to your vision may indicate.

You Can Never Seem To Get Enough Light to See Well

As you age your pupils will begin to dilate less than they did when you were younger, so you will need brighter light to see properly. If you need more light specifically for reading and close work, AMD (age related macular degeneration) or diabetic retinopathy may be obscuring the macula of your eye. An overall need for brighter light can mean that cataracts are reducing the light, which enters your eye. Fortunately, cataracts can be easily removed.

Double Vision

Double vision can originate in either your eye, or your brain. There are a number of common eye conditions that can cause double vision including:

- Dry eye
- Keratoconus
- Cataracts
- Corneal dystrophies

However, double vision can also be a sign of an underlying heath condition that may be serious and require immediate attention. Double vision can be a symptom of:

- Stroke
- Brain injury
- Aneurysm
- Brain tumor
- Diabetes
- High blood pressure
- Meningitis
- Multiple sclerosis

If you have long-term double vision, recurring double vision, or a sudden onset of severe double vision, you should never ignore these symptoms. See your doctor or ophthalmologist right away.

As we will discuss later in the book, there are certain vitamins, minerals, and herbs (Vitamin A, caretenoids, eyebright, bilberry, etc) that may delay some of the normal aging process of vision.

Hearing

As we age, there is a loss in the ability to hear high frequencies, and consonants. As a result, elderly people can have a problem with normal conversation. This type of hearing problem can often be helped with the use of a hearing aid.

What surprises many people is that some hearing loss is more commonly the result of wax that is impacted in your external ear canal, an infection in your middle ear, or degeneration of aspects of your inner ear, which is called presbycusis.

Presbycusis is a common condition in those who are over the age of 65, as a result of years of exposure to noise, and a number of different ear infections. The new cause of hearing loss will most likely be from loud iPods, cell phones, and excessive noise in auto sound systems.

These are the most common causes of hearing loss in the elderly, but of course, there are other potential causes for hearing loss.

Medications

As we age, the metabolism of medications and their absorption is affected. There are several factors that affect the absorption, and elimination of drugs from the body.

These include:

- Increased body fat
- Decreased glomerular filtration rate (kidney function),
- Reduced hepatic blood flow (liver function),
- Reduced small bowel surface area
- Reduced total muscle mass.

Obviously taking different drugs at the same time can also affect the absorption and metabolism of certain medications.

If you do not drink sufficient fluids, you drink too much alcohol, and/or you smoke, you could suffer changes in the absorption of your medication. Certain metabolic systems function less efficiently when one is older.

For example, the beta adrenergic system becomes less sensitive so that an increase in medication is necessary to obtain the same effect. Older people can also be more sensitive to certain drugs than their younger counterparts. For example, psychoactive drugs such as diazepam or hypnotics (sleeping medication) can require smaller dosages as one ages.

Aging and Drug Interactions

There are four major drug concerns that can affect the ageing body. In order of significance they are:

1. Decreased elimination of the drug from the body allowing the drug to have more effect on various body systems for a longer time.

2. Decreased hepatic (liver) metabolism of the drug allowing the substance to act differently than it was originally designed to.

3. Altered distribution of the drug in various body compartments permits the drug to have effects that were not intended in some body areas, while at the same time it does not allow the drug to 'do its thing' in other parts of the body.

4. Altered absorption from the stomach, intestines, under the tongue, etc., not permitting the drug to get into the body system to again 'do its thing'.

All of these concerns are a reality in our modern world. For here, it seems there's nothing graceful about physiologically ageing. Most of us want to hang onto our youthfulness forever, never thinking about ageing or the ageing process, which scares many. This book is packed full of information on how to age naturally, and in a healthy manner that leaves you feeling young for your age and looking great too!

The Kidneys

As people age the majority will experience a decrease in renal (kidney) function, which includes decreased blood to the kidney, smaller kidneys and decreased filtration function in the kidney.

Therefore, the elimination of a drug via the kidney may need a decrease in a drug's dosage to avoid dangerous accumulation of potentially harmful active compounds in the body.

The Liver

Liver metabolizing capacities decrease with age. Many commonly prescribed drugs are metabolized (broken down) in the liver to create the active ingredient that is necessary for the function of the drug or herb.

The metabolic process often involves an enzyme called cytochrome P450 and it is particularly vulnerable to toxicity from drugs that induce or inhibit the P450 isoenzymes.

There are even some common foods, such as grapefruit juice that can inactivate a common isoenzyme in the gastrointestinal tract. This then increases the unmetabolized concentration of certain drugs like Buspar, Tegretol, Valium, Cozaar, Mevacor, Viagra, Zocor and Halcyon to name just a few.

While it is not life threatening when a simple glass of grapefruit juice prevents a Viagra tablet from working, when it stops a blood pressure, heart failure, or seizure drug from working, one has to consider carefully what is going on.

Drug Absorption

Lastly, drug absorption is affected by age related alterations in the gastrointestinal tract {GI} (stomach, intestines, salivary glands, colon, etc).

The acid and the pH it makes can be different in the ageing body as can the amount of motility (movement) of the various parts of the GI tract. These changes can either delay or increase the absorption of common drugs.

Distribution of drugs is affected by alterations in protein binding that occur when drugs compete for the same protein-binding sites. This is more prevalent in the older population, when there is less protein-rich body mass (muscles), or less protein components in the blood like albumen. This is often due to the poor diets of older people.

Antioxidants and Their Role in Aging

Free radicals are thought to cause a wide variety of age related damage including physiological aging, arthritis, cataracts and atherosclerosis.

In various parts of this book we talk about defenses against these free radicals including scavengers such as Vitamin E, Vitamin C, beta carotene and the flavonoids.

These scavengers neutralize the free radical molecules and thus prevent some of the tissue damage that naturally occurs.

The prevention of tissue damage, and presumably the aging process, can be diminished if free radical scavengers are consumed in greater amounts, in the diet or through oral supplementation.

Of course, convincing older people, who are set in their ways, to consume more spinach, wheat germ, radishes, mushrooms, nuts, fresh fruits, raw vegetables, carrots, broccoli, mangoes and tangerines is not always the easiest thing to do but is important if, alternatively, oral supplementation with vitamins is not carried out.

There have been various studies from the National Institute of Aging in the U.S. (Dr. Richard Cutler) that indicate that as our cells age in our body, they tend to forget specifically what they're supposed to do.

According to Dr. Cutler, cells regress to a generic and generally useless form. He speculates that free radical damage to the DNA is what causes this regression. Currently, one of the most intriguing questions in free radical research is whether effective, free radical control can slow the aging process and extend one's life.

Arbitrary tests with mice and fruit flies have shown that the use of various herbs can extend the life of these animals.

- Dr. Jeremy Fields at the University of Loyola found significantly increased life span when Ayurvedic herbs were used.

- Dr. Paul Gelderloos at MIU subjected human subjects with various performance tests. Again the use of various Ayurvedic herbs showed statistically significant improvement in the groups that took the herbs in comparison to the placebo group.

This is strongly correlated with age but showed improvement in all age groups after three to six weeks. These results give positive credentials to the free radical paradigm, indicating the free radical scavenging of various herbs can improve cell functioning, and thereby improve physical/mental processes.

When Our Muscles Hurt

We all know that pains in the hands, knees, elbows, shoulders, and back are less common in young people than they are in older people, or those who have had sports injuries. Millions of people take analgesics such as aspirin and Tylenol or non-steroidal anti-inflammatory medicines such as Ibuprofen for these aches and pains.

Locally people will utilize a number of pomades and gels for local alleviation of joint aches and pains. In Europe, it is quite common for people to use anti-inflammatory gels.

Joint aches and pains are fairly common – they are just a fact of life. Lifting things in an uncomfortable way, past traumas, and past physiological disease, all contribute to joint pain. When this pain persists, it's important to have a physician make a proper diagnosis with a physical examination, X-ray and laboratory testing. With this, it can be determined as to whether there are bony joint abnormalities, muscular abnormalities or ligament strains. It can also be determined if there are infectious or other inflammatory etiologies for an arthritic phenomenon. In some individuals, a Vitamin D or calcium deficiency, particularly in aged individuals, will indicate if osteoporosis is a problem.

Allopathic medicine is highly effective in treating acute traumatic joint problems and acute muscular stains. Chronic difficulties are a horse of a different color. Chronic use of an anti-inflammatory both non-steroidal and steroidal, have significant side effects including gastric, intestinal, and others.

Consequently, with chronic joint aches and pains that are not infectious in origin, the use of various herbal preparations, both locally and internally, can create long lasting effects, without significant side effects.

- La reine des pres-elusanes capsules, d'harpagophytum (harpadol, arthrosan) are treatments that are based on herbal preparations for joint discomfort. Cats claw (Una de gato), glucosamine, condroitin sulfate, and MSM also are used for joint discomforts.

- Numerous oils are used in massage for joint pain. Ayurvedic oils have been found to be extremely effective. A mixture of essential oils such as lavender, eucalyptus, Italian helichryse, and genevrier mixed with a vegetable oil is also highly effective.

- Rhus-toxicodendron is the classical homeopathic remedy for painful joints.

- Remineralization treatments dictate that oligo elements are necessary in the cartilage, and the bony tissues to decrease inflammation (sulfur phosphorus and silica).

  When the normal balance is present and further treatment is necessary copper, cobalt, and manganese are utilized to treat joint inflammation. This type of remineralization treatment usually lasts one to two months.

Muscle Contractions

When muscles are strained, and the pain that one has results from a muscle contraction, stretch, or contusion; allopathic medicine usually uses anti-inflammatory or muscle relaxants to treat. These can be quite effective in acute traumatic experiences, and allow for rapid repair when there is significant damage.

Immobilization is sometimes necessary. This can be accomplished with various bracing or supportive elastic bandages. This practice is sometimes contraindicated when gentle range of motion of the muscle is appropriate with certain types of strains. This is where consultation with the physical therapist is often appropriate.

When there are chronic periods of cramping one needs to look at the amount of calcium that is being consumed by the individual. Often supplementation is necessary. Similarly, certain cramping conditions can be alleviated with quinine derivatives, calcium, and Vitamin B1.

Homeopathic remedies such as metallicun or dencrampem are traditionally used for cramping. In the oligo element method, a deficiency of potassium is often indicated as the etiology of cramping and muscular pain.

Local treatments of sprained muscles can be obtained through anti-inflammatory gels and creams, massage with essential oils, and massages with Ayurvedic oils. Certain creative, healing techniques have also been indicated in treatment of muscle strains. Essential oils with camphor, eucalyptus, and pine are utilized for these muscle spasms.

French Thalo Therapy

Thalo Therapy (thalassotherapy). The term thalo therapy originated in French speaking Europe. It has been in vogue in Europe for many centuries in many different forms. It is also associated with the term thermalisme, or thermal therapy. The latter tends to involve more of the medical treatments, which are specific for specific conditions.

'Taking the baths' has been popular in Europe for centuries both in French and German speaking areas. Many resorts, thermal therapy baths, treatment centers, and spas have flourished on and off for many hundreds of years. In the 1990's thermal therapy was restricted to a few rather sparse centers.

What has replaced thermal therapy has been the lassale therapy, which tends to be more fashionable and acceptable to those with sufficient funds, but at the same time have some mild medical condition treated.

Although there is a list of maladies that have claimed to be treated in some of these resorts, the validation of disease treatment regimes hold some large questions as to their effectiveness; and in the end, one can compare the effects to the placebo effect. Placebo aside, there are many of thalo therapies and thermalisme treatments, which do hold therapeutic benefit, when they are <u>added</u> to other regimens, and for certain conditions, they can be beneficial.

So what is new in thermal therapy, since the 1990's? Statistics show that 44% of all people seeking thermal therapy are utilizing it to recuperate after a period of difficulty in their lives particularly with stress, fatigue or other anxieties.

In a traditional thermal therapy treatment, a person will check into a center for one to two weeks and expect to have four treatments per day, regulated diet, and some form of evaluation by either a therapist or a visiting physician.

Often times, treatment with physiotherapy exercises, hydrotherapy and a variety of baths, saunas, steam baths, muscle building and other exercises are all presented to the visitor.

Traditionally, a few of the treatments are included in a global package with the exception of medical examinations, laboratory examinations, or osteopathic treatments. This of course depends on the center in which somebody has chosen a visit. Belo therapy units are always associated with institutes of beauty, which will carry out various treatments on skin and hair. Again these may or may not be included in a package. For many medical and psychological conditions, just the caring attention of another human and having restful, stress-reducing treatments, in and of itself, can be therapeutic.

Smoother Skin, Fewer Wrinkles

In the aging process, for those that don't like to see wrinkles on their face, there are many products on the market that claim to decrease premature aging of the skin, and the elimination of wrinkles. Some of these products are excellent and do what they claim while others are totally bogus.

There are also products, which can fill in wrinkles with collagen (animal protein) ingredients. An ongoing dermatological rage, of course, is Botox. This product paralyzes the small muscles in the face to eliminate the appearance of the wrinkles on a temporary basis.

There are also various products that when applied on a regular basis will help eliminate facial wrinkles and smooth the skin. These formulations have two basic ingredients: retinol and Vitamin C and they are topically applied.

When these products are applied in a cream base, they act to reduce the appearance of fine lines and wrinkles, improve texture and tone of skin, and refine the size of natural pores. The overall effect of this dermatological phenomenon is to have smoother, wrinkle free skin.

Of course, there are innumerable products, which claim to be better than the other one. These products can help, if used along with a nutritious diet and appropriate vitamin supplementation, which of course assists the overall health of the skin.

To apply retinol and Vitamin A, you need to be careful not to get it in the eye or near the delicate skin around your eyes. If these products do come in contact with your eye(s), you need to wash the eye out thoroughly to remove the product and seek medical care.

When the product is applied, you will often experience a tingling and light redness of the skin. This is a normal reaction to these products. If this redness continues, one must decrease the amount of applications to alternate days, for instance. If the products create a more prominent or continued redness (erythema), one must seek medical advice and stop using the product.

When looking at a product that claims to remove wrinkles the ingredients that you might like to see that product include a moisturizing agent, water based, glycerin, retinol (Vitamin A.), tocopheryl acetate (Vitamin E.), ascorbic acid (Vitamin C), and a variety of essential oils and herbs. Other ingredients include the use of Neem oil, (a traditional treatment for all skin problems in India–and the claim that it is the reason all Indian women have such beautiful skin). Commercial products with Neem oil may smell less pungent than the pure oil, but obviously less effective too.

For those with significant scarring and injury to their facial skin, there are also some laser technologies, which are somewhat successful in removing significant pathologies. Like other products, the claims may exceed the actual results.

There are a multitude of products that claim to help reduce scars' appearance. This is not an endorsement of these products, but here are a few products that have seen okay results:

Scarprin

Scarprin is made of 100% silicone gel. Multiple clinical studies support silicone based scar products as being more effective than other ingredients (such as onion extract and certain vitamins) some of which actually cause harm to the scar. In fact, silicone has been widely used for scar reduction since the 1980's and has been used in numerous clinical studies, all of which found it to be effective for minimizing the appearance of most scars, including keloids, acne scars and burn scars.

Dermatix

Although the silicone formulation in this product appears to be quite effective at treating scars, its inclusion of a Vitamin C ester may reduce its potential effectiveness.

While Vitamin C is known to reduce pigmentation and brighten the appearance of the skin, it also promotes the formation of collagen, which is the primary component of scar tissue. Additionally, studies have shown that the most dramatic results of silicone are achieved from undiluted formulations.

Bio Oil

Bio Oil has been clinically tested and appears to be somewhat effective at reducing the appearance of scars. It uses mineral oil as its main ingredient. Bio Oil claims to help improve the appearance of scars, stretch marks, and uneven skin tone with the use of PurCellin Oil.

According to one clinical trial on Bio Oil, 65% of the subjects tested exhibited an improvement in the appearance of their scars within 4 weeks. However, this one test was only conducted on Caucasians and was not scientifically validated.

The Aging Brain

As we age, our short-term memory and a variety of other changes occur in the brain. There are many studies that have tried to determine exactly what happens when the brain malfunctions in its aging years.

Various forms of dementia, including Alzheimer's disease, occur in older age. There are a variety of things that can be done to diminish aging brain function, including the use of antioxidants, and the use of a variety of foods.

Maintaining the responsibility of a job, even a simple job, will often keep the brain active. If having a job is not what you want to do, stay active mentally with various exercises for the brain. Mental exercises are vital in delaying the deterioration seen with normal aging. Many of these brain exercises are very simple but are useful in maintaining brain function.

Examples of Some Simple but Effective Brain Exercises

1. Looking at a picture for a few seconds then writing down as many details as can be remembered about that picture.

2. Looking at an old photograph and trying to reconstruct the events depicted in the photo.

3. Complete crossword puzzles, and brain games like Soduku.

4. Play mind games on your computer like Tetris or Bejeweled.

5. Choosing a controversial topic and arguing the opposite opinion to your own view.

6. Writing down five unusual uses of an everyday object.

12 Ways to Keep Your Brain Young

Harvard Medical School says "Every brain changes with age, and mental function changes along with it. Mental decline is common, and it's one of the most feared consequences of aging. But cognitive impairment is not inevitable. Here are 12 ways you can help reduce your risk of age-related memory loss."

1. Get Mental Stimulation

Through research with mice and humans, doctors suspect that brainy activities stimulate new connections between nerve cells and may even help the brain generate new cells, developing neurological "plasticity" and building up a functional reserve that provides a hedge against future cell loss.

Any mentally stimulating activity should help to build up your brain. Read, take courses, and try "mental gymnastics," such as word puzzles or math problems Experiment with things that require manual dexterity as well as mental effort, such as drawing, painting, and other crafts.

2. Get Physical Exercise

Research shows that using your muscles may also help your mind. Animals who exercise regularly increase the number of tiny blood vessels that bring oxygen-rich blood to the region of the brain that is responsible for thought.

Exercise also spurs the development of new nerve cells and increases the connections between brain cells (synapses). This results in brains that are more efficient, plastic, and adaptive, which translates into, better performance in aging animals.

Exercise also lowers blood pressure, improves cholesterol levels, fights diabetes, and reduces mental stress, all of which can help your brain as well as your heart.

3. Improve Your Diet

Good nutrition can help your mind as well as your body. Here are some specifics:

- **Keep your calories in check**. In both animals and humans, a reduced caloric intake has been linked to a lower risk of mental decline in old age.

- **Eat the right foods.** That means reducing your consumption of saturated fat and cholesterol from animal sources and of trans-fatty acids from partially hydrogenated vegetable oils (fried food in particular).

- **Remember your Bs.** Three B vitamins, folic acid, B6, and B12, can help lower your homocysteine levels, high levels of which have been linked to an increased risk of dementia. Fortified cereal, other grains, and leafy green vegetables are good sources of B vitamins.

4. Improve Your Blood Pressure

High blood pressure in midlife increases the risk of cognitive decline in old age. Use lifestyle modification and medication if recommended by your doctor, to keep your pressure as low as possible. Stay lean, exercise regularly, limit your alcohol, reduce stress, and eat right.

5. Improve Your Blood Sugar

Diabetes is a significant risk factor for dementia. You can fight diabetes by eating right, adding chromium your diet, exercising regularly, and staying lean. But if your blood sugar stays high, you'll need medication to achieve good control.

6. Improve Your Cholesterol

High levels of LDL ("bad") cholesterol increase the risk of dementia, as do low levels of HDL ("good") cholesterol. Diet, exercise, weight control, and avoiding tobacco will go a long way toward improving your cholesterol levels. But if you need more help, ask your doctor about statin medications or the natural Plant Sterols.

7. Consider Low-Dose Aspirin

Observational studies suggest that long-term use of low-dose aspirin (81 mg) may reduce the risk of dementia by 10%-55%. It's hopeful information, but it's preliminary. Experts are not ready to recommend aspirin specifically for dementia.

8. Avoid Tobaccos

Avoid tobacco in all its forms.

9. Don't Abuse Alcohol

Excessive drinking is a major risk factor for dementia. If you choose to drink, limit yourself to a tablespoon or small glass of wine a day. But if you use alcohol responsibly, you may actually reduce your risk of dementia. Five studies have linked low-dose red wine with a reduced risk of dementia in older adults.

10. Care for Your Emotions

People who are anxious, depressed, sleep-deprived, or exhausted tend to score poorly on cognitive function tests. Poor scores don't necessarily predict an increased risk of cognitive decline in old age, but good mental health and restful sleep are certainly important goals.

11. Protect Your Head

You may be surprised to learn that moderate to severe head injuries early in life increase the risk of cognitive impairment in old age. Concussions increase risk by a factor of 10.

12. Build Social Networks

Strong social ties have been associated with lower blood pressure and longer life expectancies. Collect friends.

While most of these tips are well known by health conscious people, and certainly discussed throughout this book, we thought we'd also include what Harvard Medical School has to say.

Aging and the Mind Body Experience

Modern medicine has recently begun to find objective evidence to support what most doctors once knew from their own practice – feeling good could make you well. We all recognize that stress, tension, anxiety, fear, sadness, and disappointment can all lead to physical illness.

For centuries, physicians and healers only had mild natural medications, along with a reassuring bedside manner, to heal their patients. From shamans to family doctors, these healers knew if the patient felt comforted and encouraged (providing the disease was not over-powering), would do better and eventually end up healed.

Unfortunately, with managed care, national medicine, and other socialized economic health care systems, the time necessary to reassure patients is not always available to the physician and healer. There has been a great deal of research done, which confirms that the old healing touch of the physician is better medicine.

We know that stress affects mental functioning, and in turn affects physiological functioning because stress creates free radicals in abundance and changes the physiology of the cardiovascular system and the endocrine system.

We also know that stress affects our health, and our aging process. Furthermore, we know that severe mental depression can cause suppression of the immune system.

Similarly, we have been able to show that a positive mental state, love, laughter, and support groups can increase the survival time for patients with cancer and various otherwise terminal diseases. Many books have been written about these relationships, and the term: mind body medicine, has developed as a nineties term.

How Does This Work?

The part of the brain that regulates emotions has a close physiological connection between feelings in the functioning of the body. This network is called the limbic system, which includes the pituitary gland, the hypothalamus, (which is the body's central regulatory switch board) and a variety of other nerve fibers in the small area at the base of the brain.

The hypothalamus regulates temperature, thirst, blood sugar levels, hunger, growth, sleeping, and waking, and emotions such as anger and happiness. Just underneath the hypothalamus is the pituitary gland, the body's master endocrine control system. This emits various hormones that control the activities of many other glands in the body.

So if there is a change in emotions it creates a new mix of molecules, which transforms the functioning of the physical body through this

Limbic system. Stimuli coming from the limbic region of the brain cause the Hypothalamus to release a wide variety of Neuropeptides.

In turn, these Neuropeptides stimulate specific hormones from the pituitary gland, and the specific activity in all the other endocrine glands including the thymus and adrenal glands. Specific chemical messengers are released when emotions raise certain physiological actions.

The biochemical output of these systems is changed on a regular basis, based on the mood of the individual. In short, contents of your conscious behavior, alters the physiology of your body here and now. Your actions and your mood can directly affect various cells in the body such as lymphocytes.

Research has shown that these lymphocytes or special white blood cells can respond molecularly to messages created by the neuropeptides directly produced from the hypothalamus.

But there is a reverse to the hypothalamus regulating the body cells in that some of the chemicals created by the lymphocytes (interleukins) can directly affect the hypothalamus, because of receptors that are sensitive to them.

As a result, the chemical messages from the immune system (lymphocytes) can modulate the nervous system function, and the mental state through the hypothalamus.

This two way communication network between the brain and the immune system evident in various moods, the nervous system in general, and the immune system are tied together in this network, and easily explain the reason that mood has a definite physiological effect on the human body.

Negative emotions can depress the immune system through this mechanism and allow the patient to become sicker. Similarly, positive thoughts, love, support, and a good bedside manner from the doctor can stimulate the production of the neuropeptides that help the immune system function.

Certain herbs that have been used for centuries in India and China have been shown to encourage the body's natural production of endorphins, enkephalins, and other natural painkillers. Some of these herbs have also been shown to increase the positive functioning of the immune system.

Similarly, there are certain herbs that have been used for centuries that have a calming effect on the nervous system. It has been shown that this calming effect influences the positive emotions, and thereby influences the immune system so has healing affects in several different ways.

Certain herbs have been shown to decrease substance P. This substance P is triggered by pain and associated with various inflammations in the body. Other herbs have been shown to increase the levels of serotonin, a neuro-transmitter associated with depression when it is decreased in the body.

Consequently utilizing some of these herbs can decrease depression, inflammation and pain. These herbs are ancient combinations of various individual herbs that contain natural vitamins, polyphenols, antioxidants, and bioflavonoids.

Although it is often necessary to utilize individual components in higher quantities for certain diseases, the general feeling now is that by using these herbal combinations, one gets significantly more benefits by the natural synergism that these combinations provide.

Although we can measure certain improvements utilizing these herbal combinations, with regard to therapeutic means, the improvement in the physical health and mental well-being of individuals is significant in many immeasurable ways.

'All You Need is Love'

As John Lennon said, 'all you need is love'. Love of yourself and others comes thru to the surface. Looking beautiful comes from within. When you take good care of yourself (with proper diet, exercise, and a good skin care regimen including sun protection), you feel good about that internally, and it will show on the outside, too.

We Are All Getting Older

No matter how badly you want the aging process to stop, it's never going to happen. However, you now have some tools available that can help you slow the aging process, and keep you looking and feeling younger than your birth years. Then again, what really is an age other than a number?

Some people are in their 30's and feel like they are in their 60's, while others are in their 80's and feel like they are in their 60's. What age do you want to feel?

CHAPTER 5
MEDICAL CONDITIONS

Everything in our bodies is in a state of flux. We tend to think that our bodies are very stable. After all, we see our body in the mirror on a daily basis, and it doesn't appear to change significantly from day to day. In reality, our bodies are constantly changing.

Our bodies are nothing like a piece of furniture or a statue. They are much more like a river that has various aspects of nutrients, water, energy, intelligence, and structure flowing by on a minute-by-minute basis.

As teenagers, our perception of our bodies changed as we grew hair in various parts of our body, the shape of our body changed, our voices changed, we became sexually mature, and mentally our thought processes matured and changed–for most of us.

In middle age, we noticed similar kinds of changes – changes in the color, consistency, and presence of hair; the growth of hair in places we never thought possible; further changes to the shape of our bodies, with gravity taking its toll; changes in sexual activity; and changes in vision, hearing, etc.

Unfortunately, as we get older the list goes on. Don't worry, there are many recommendations in this book about ways to modify those changes, keeping you looking and feeling younger.

If we look at the physiology of the human body, we note that almost all aspects of the human body change. This is based upon the cellular structure of our body organs and fluids. Our red blood cells change every twenty-one days, and every five days we acquire a new stomach lining.

Our skin changes every five weeks, while the bones that make up our skeleton change every three months. And even though the deposits of fat cells appear to never change, in reality they are exchanged every twenty-one days.

A perfectly normal individual can expect 98% of the physical structure of the human body to have been replaced, or changed in some manner every year. Unfortunately, certain diseases will change those rates of change and they do not allow the replacement of certain tissues.

Arthritis

Arthritis is a chronic disease, which affects both young and old. There are two kinds of arthritis, rheumatoid arthritis, and osteoarthritis. Arthritis means, "joint inflammation." Inflammation is the body's natural reaction to injury or disease, and it can result in pain, stiffness, and swelling. When the inflammation lasts for a long time it can cause tissue damage.

A joint is described as a place where two or more bones come together. The joint is covered with cartilage, which provides cushion to the bones, and allows the painless movement of the joint.

The inside of the joint is lined with synovium, which is a thin film of tissue. The synovium produces a synovial fluid, a slippery fluid that reduces friction to the joint and helps to keep it stable.

When there is arthritis, the area surrounding the joint becomes inflamed, leading to pain, and stiffness that can make movements difficult.

Unfortunately, the most prevalent form of arthritis is osteoarthritis, which usually begins around age fifty for most individuals. Some individuals rank this as the number one health problem in people over age forty-five. It is recognized that by the time an individual is sixty-five, half of all North Americans will have some form of arthritis. If you have injured any particular joint or injured other tissues affecting the joint, like muscles, the stresses on that joint are unusual and you may well end up with arthritis long before age 50.

In 1997, nearly forty million Americans suffered from arthritis. Because of the baby boomers, the Center of Disease Control and Prevention estimates that, by the year 2020, nearly sixty million Americans will suffer from arthritis.

There are many allopathic medical treatments that have been utilized for the treatment and control of arthritis. Unfortunately, many of these only control the symptoms of arthritis, and not the cause. Changes in diet and exercise are considered the most effective methods of changing the outcome of osteoarthritis.

Rheumatoid arthritis is a horse of a slightly different color. It is a much more aggressive disease than osteoarthritis and has many more systemic effects than osteoarthritis.

In this book we will mostly refer to osteoarthritis rather than rheumatoid arthritis.

Treatments for "the other arthritides" have changed over the years. For example, various anti-cancer drugs (Methotrexate) have been used to control rheumatoid arthritis and its symptoms. A variety of treatments are utilized to treat yet another type of arthritis, which results from an infection from the Borrelia Burgdorferi tick-otherwise known as Lyme disease. Similarly, the utilization of Interferon to treat rheumatoid arthritis has not proved as successful as originally hoped in treating this type of arthritis. Using the immune system molecules such as Interferon in conjunction with ultra potent chemotherapeutic agents such as Cisplatin, are now being used to treat not only cancers, but in an attempt to also treat arthritis. Again, these drugs have significant affects on other body systems and are not gentle in any way, shape, or form.

The large class of drugs known as non-steroidal anti-inflammatory drugs (NSAID) is used for all kinds of arthritis. These drugs are usually helpful in treating some of the symptoms of osteoarthritis. They have not been shown to modify the overall course of this disease.

Exercise Improves Arthritis

One finding over the years has shown that certain exercises do help improve the outcome for people with arthritis. This applies to not only osteoarthritis but also rheumatoid arthritis.

As long as a person "listens to his/her body," exercise is very helpful. If, for example, a joint is hot and inflamed and painful, that joint needs to be rested. With the arthritic patient, there is no gain in the adage of 'no pain no gain'. One needs to mobilize the joints, and once a flair-up is over one can slowly build up to more physical activity utilizing that joint.

While a joint is inflamed, or painful, other exercise can be utilized such as water therapy, and the overall positive benefits of exercise will help relieve the problems with the inflamed joints.

As long as a patient protects their joints, they can be active in whatever activity that they chose. Each of us has an activity that is more suited to our body type and demeanor. Some people are built as runners, others as swimmers, still others as bicyclists. Participating in certain exercises that their body is not designed for can damage certain bodies.

Most people can exercise at 60% to 80% of their maximum heart rate on a regular basis. Not only can they enjoy increased cardiovascular fitness, they can improve their joint and immune function, which are just some of the positive benefits of exercise. Strengthening, aerobic, and flexibility exercises can help ease pain, improve function, and improve the patients overall feeling of well-being.

Extracting data from the Framingham study has shown that excess weight can induce, or aggravate arthritis; and that losing weight before symptoms occur can reduce the risk of developing osteoarthritis in certain joints such as the knees and ankles.

Since the Framingham study, in 1992, others have implicated that excess weight can be a contributing factor to osteoarthritis and that losing excess weight can not only decrease symptoms of osteoarthritis but also help prevent the condition in the first place.

Treating Arthritis With Relaxation

Relaxation has been shown to be extremely beneficial to the treatment and prevention of arthritis. By resting in a comfortable, secluded spot and practicing relaxation or meditation techniques, you will reduce your muscle tension, lower your heart rate, and reduce your blood pressure. It has also shown to chemically relax the body so that conditions such as arthritis are minimized.

Similarly, after a full day's activity, one must rest the joints. It is important that one's daily routine is a mixture of activity and rest, rather than all one or the other.

Fibromyalgia

Fibromyalgia is a term, which many allopathic physicians feel has no basis in science. Unfortunately many unscrupulous individuals latch onto the fact that fibromyalgia does not have specific science behind it and make it a 'diagnosis' for which they charge great sums of money to "cure". There have been various fibromyalgia studies measuring the serum level of Somatomedin C. This is a hormone that is secreted principally during stage four of sleep, in some patients. However, the results of these studies and many others trying to define what fibromyalgia really is have been contradictory.

Some studies have shown that sufferers of fibromyalgia have lower levels of this hormone, where as other studies have shown that there is no difference in fibromyalgia patients, and control subjects. Interestingly, these studies have consistently shown that there are more disturbed sleep patterns among individuals with fibromyalgia than among the controlled subjects. This leaves many scientists believing that fibromyalgia is more a psychosomatic and/ or a psychological disease than a physical one.

Chronic Fatigue

Chronic fatigue is another medical condition, which has great debate in both allopathic and holistic worlds. The word fatigue refers to a condition of cells or organs that have undergone excessive activity, resulting in a loss of power or capacity to respond to stimulation. True fatigue implies that the physiology of your body has gone beyond being merely 'tired'. If we speak of exhausting the body, it implies that we are draining strength, or that a supply of energy is gone.

Unlike some other medical diagnoses such as diabetes or certain skin rashes, fatigue is less easy to define. Furthermore, because of its elusive nature many people misinterpret the feeling of fatigue.

If after only sleeping two hours, you get up and you feel tired you are perfectly normal. If you slept a normal night and did a regular amount of work during the day, and felt tired, you also would be perfectly normal.

However, if you sleep a normal period of time, you don't have any other serious medical problems, and you still cannot do a reasonable amount of work during the day because of feeling fatigued, then you might be suffering from a more chronic form of fatigue, or some other yet undiagnosed medical or psychological condition.

If your body is chronically fatigued, there is something wrong. There may be something physical, psychological, or emotional wrong. There are various kinds of fatigue ranging from minimal to severe.

Some call being tired all the time chronic fatigue, and the most severe form of this is labeled by some as "Chronic Fatigue Immune Dysfunction Syndrome" or simply "Chronic Fatigue Syndrome" by some practitioners.

This delineation is not universally accepted in the medical world. In this book, we will refer to the problem of fatigue as it encompasses all aspects of medically debilitating levels of fatigue.

To be medically debilitating a person has to experience a 50% loss of activity over a six-month period from a new onset of fatigue that started over that period of time. Generally, fatigue patients will also demonstrate other medical and emotional problems.

For the patient with significant fatigue, there are several areas that one first looks at to determine the cause of this problem.

- How much stress exists?
- How much sleep do you get?
- How good is that sleep?
- Is it a drug induced sleep or is it naturally occurring?
- Do you have periods of depression?
- How are your relationships with others at home and in the job?
- What is your diet?
- What medications do you take?
- Do you smoke?
- How much alcohol do you consume?
- Do you take any other illicit drugs?
- Are you able to carry out regular activities of daily living? For example, preparing meals, cleaning house, attending your job, performing at your job, performing normal duties in a family situation, etc.

Fatigue has many faces, and there are many people who feel tired all the time but don't know why. Unfortunately, their lack of energy does not permit them to intellectually evaluate why they are tired.

Then there are others who understand that they have a problem, but are unwilling to accept medical or psychological help or lifestyle changes that are necessary to solve their particular problem.

The Type A personality that pushes way too hard is often the person that refuses to slow down, until such time as a catastrophic medical event happens. We define seven basic causes of fatigue. They are:

- ☑ Medical illnesses
- ☑ Thyroid disease
- ☑ Depression
- ☑ Severe stress
- ☑ Emotional dysfunction,
- ☑ Poor nutrition
- ☑ A variety of sleep disorders.

Dietary Malfunctions

In many instances, fatigue is due to a variety of dietary malfunctions. This can be caused by:

- ☑ Specific nutrients missing from the diet
- ☑ An excess of foods or nutrients, which adversely affect the body
- ☑ A global situation of malnutrition such as one sees in starving individuals in third world countries.

Similarly, people with certain diseases will have the inability to absorb proper amounts of food because of mechanical or biochemical reasons. Pernicious anemia is one such condition where the body is missing Vitamin B12. The surgical procedures performed to staple or band the stomach for significant weight loss, can lead to nutritional deficiencies.

In these situations, one is unable to absorb other nutrients from the food, which results in the red blood cells not getting their iron, so they can rebuild. As a result, the person ends up anemic. With this condition, a person is quite fatigued.

In the normal individual, the body allows you to process nutritious food and store the energy released from it. When the body is working properly, and you need the energy at a time other than when you're eating the meal, you simply tap into the body's storage sites.

With diet there are many potential theories of how a poor diet causes fatigue. While nutritional and medical disorders often overlap, poor nutrition is a common culprit behind fatigue.

Fatigue can also be caused by too much food. Obese people tend to use up excessive amounts of energy in carrying their increased body weight. There are also other aspects to obesity, which can contribute to a fatigue syndrome.

Medical Illnesses

There are many medical conditions, which can be associated with fatigue. These range anywhere from the common cold to seasonal allergies on one end of the spectrum to severe debilitating diseases such as Multiple Sclerosis on the other. Various viral diseases have been linked to fatigue type syndromes also.

It was quite popular several years ago to relate chronic fatigue to Epstein–Barr virus infection. This was also known as yuppie flu, Myalgic Encephalomyelitis and Chronic Fatigue Immune Deficiency Syndrome. Current research has not linked any fatigue syndromes to the Epstein–Barr virus although initial studies did find some correlation.

In summary, fatigue syndromes can be from valid medical and physiological conditions as we have described above. Unfortunately, there are other individuals who have no medical reason to be fatigued but latch onto the diagnosis of 'chronic fatigue' as an escape from life's responsibilities and stresses. These individuals would be better served by getting needed psychological/counseling treatments that could help them to lead happy and productive lives.

Sleep Disorders

The main causes of fatigue include sleep disorders, poor nutrition, specific medical illnesses, depression, and stress or emotion.

Basically, if sleep disorders are the reason you are chronically fatigued, it is that you are not sleeping well or long enough. It might be something as simple as too much noise or light, an uncomfortable bed, or a sleep disorder such as sleep apnea or narcolepsy.

If you have a condition such as arthritis that makes your muscles or joints ache, this can also contribute to the inability to sleep well and or sleep at all.

Similarly, if you have a bladder or prostate problem that requires you to get up frequently during the night to go to the bathroom, you will be unable to sleep extended periods of time. Excessive drinking of alcohol, and caffeine containing beverages can also contribute to poor sleep as can the use of other medications including diet pills etc.

There are many studies that indicate that proper sleep needs to occur, for the well-being of the individual. For the body to receive proper rest, various biorhythms need to be completed. Failure to have sufficient periods of sleep with alpha rhythms or beta rhythms can lead to fatigue.

People who travel from different time zones on a regular basis and or are assigned to rotating shift changes at work can also suffer from circadian dysrhythmias, which can contribute to fatigue.

Depression

Depression is a condition where either emotional or physiological imbalances have occurred.

This is to be differentiated from simple reactional depression such as the blues one has following loss of a job, loss of a loved one, etc. This type of temporary depression is a very specific post loss depression that usually resolves itself in time with proper adaptation to the loss and the grieving process. This does not usually lead to fatigue.

Other forms of depression, which are more long standing, are the kind that will lead to fatigue. There is significant evidence that serotonin (an enzyme found in the brain) levels have a great deal to do with the presence or absence of depression.

Many allopathic drugs are now designed to insure that the level of serotonin is maintained in the brain, which has been found to be very successful in eliminating the symptoms of depression and its results in fatigue.

Stress

Stress is a normal part of human existence. There has been no definition of stress that everyone accepts. Scientifically, stress can refer to the hypothalamic-pituitary-adrenal axis or stimulation of the sympathetic nervous system and adrenalin secretion in the "fight or flight" response.

Everyone defines stress differently. Probably the most common is, "physical, mental, or emotional strain or tension". Stress is a subjective phenomenon that differs for each of us. There is no definition of stress that all scientists agree on.

Hans Selye, a famous Swiss physician, was one of the first to define stress and many of its ramifications. He delineated stress and distress as being very important. Regular stress, which keeps us going during the day and motivates us to carry on with life, is referred to as good stress.

The original definition of stress by Hans Selye, who coined the term as it is presently used, was, "the non-specific response of the body to any demand for change".

Another popular definition of stress is, "a condition or feeling experienced when a person perceives that demands exceed the personal and social resources the individual is able to mobilize."

Most people consider the definition of stress to be something that causes distress. However, stress is not always harmful since increased stress results in increased productivity and creativity.

A definition of stress should also embrace this type of healthy stress, which is usually ignored when you ask someone about his or her definition of stress. Any definition of stress should also include good stress, or eustress.

For example, winning a road race is just as stressful as losing. A passionate kiss and contemplating what might follow is stressful, but hardly the same as the thought of having root canal work done.

All definitions of stress, should similarly explain the difference between eustress and distress.

Distress can come from psychological causes, such as the death of a loved one; sleep deprivation, work stress, marital stress, economic stress, etc. Distress can also come from physical stress like; overwork without sufficient rest, sun exposure, chemical or radiation exposure, drugs, cigarette smoking, alcohol, etc.

In the biopsychosocial definition of stress, the outside environment makes up one aspect and the other aspect consists of physiological and biochemical factors in our body.

This theory of stress says that it is the interaction between these two that causes stress. Some of the physical reactions experienced during stress include hypertension, palpitations, arrhythmias, headaches, gastrointestinal problems, skin complaints, etc.

Selye created the word, stressor, to distinguish between stimulus and response. In the end, he suggested that the best definition of stress was "the rate of wear and tear on the body".

There are many ways of dealing with stress and eliminating distress from our bodies. We will cover various methods of dealing with stress at a later point in this book.

Stress Symptoms

Losing interest in doing enjoyable activities can be one of the first signs of stress, which include being short tempered, bored, nervous, or being ineffective in handling things that previously were handled easily.

Fatigue, anger, unexplained insomnia, and depression indicate that stress is becoming more entrenched in one's lifestyle with some of the following physiological responses:

- ☑ High blood pressure
- ☑ Gastrointestinal problems
- ☑ Palpitations of the heart
- ☑ Headaches
- ☑ Backaches and other muscle aches

When heart disease, chronic skin disorders, ulcers, stroke, and more significant psychological problems are evident, stress may be at the root of this.

Environmental influences from childhood may also have some influence on adult age stress. Regardless of what definition of stress you find relevant, reducing stress can provide considerable health rewards.

Hypoglycemia

Sugars are an essential fuel in the human body, and without them, we do not generate energy and we are not alert. A certain level of sugar in the blood is what is necessary for alertness.

If that sugar is being stored in the liver, or elsewhere in the body, it is of no help to the organs that need it directly from the blood stream. Consequently when the blood sugar level drops it can cause a multitude of symptoms including physical and mental lethargy.

Mid-afternoon is a common time for individuals to experience low blood sugar levels. This usually happens after a large meal at lunchtime.

When your blood sugar is low, various organs will show a variety of symptoms. When the brain doesn't get sufficient blood sugar, it is difficult to concentrate, and one can be irritable or depressed. One might also have cravings for certain foods including sugary foods.

The proper diet is essential for people who have suffered from hypoglycemia. The ideal diet is the "Chicken Diet." This means you eat small amounts of food on a regular basis, particularly complex carbohydrates such as whole grains. It earned its name, because you eat much as a chicken does–you peck at food all day long.

This allows the blood sugar to never drop too low so it does not go into the danger zone where you would then experience symptoms. For people who experience hypoglycemia often get use to eating foods that are high in slow releasing sugar such as whole grains, proteins such as nuts, fish, and vegetables at least every two to three hours.

Chromium in several forms, including the Plycnicotinate form, is helpful in stabilizing blood sugar. This product is also helpful in stabilizing the blood sugar of diabetics.

Gallstones

According to Michael Smith MD, eating monounsaturated and polyunsaturated fat lowered the risk of gallstones.

A new study shows eating more olive oil, and less butter may help reduce the risk of gallstones. Researchers found that men/women who ate a diet high in monounsaturated or polyunsaturated fats, such as those found in plant and olive oils, were 18% less likely to develop gallstones than people who ate the least of these types of fat.

Other studies have also shown that the type of fat people eat may affect their risk of developing gallstones. For example, diets high in saturated fats, such as those found in red meat and whole milk, may promote the formation of gallstones.

This study adds: "in addition to keeping saturated fats to a minimum, eating a diet rich in unsaturated fats (polyunsaturated fats, and monounsaturated fats) may further reduce a risk of gallstones."

Gallstones are caused by changes in bile, which is a fluid produced by the liver to help digest food. Bile contains a mixture of cholesterol, fats, and other substances. When changes in bile occur, such as too much cholesterol, it can cause bile to crystallize and form gallstones. Cholesterol gallstones account for nearly 80% to 90% of all gallstones removed from middle-aged adults.

The Type of Fat Matters

In the study, published in a recent issue of the *Annals of Internal Medicine*, researchers compared the diets of more than 45,000 men between the ages of 40 and 75. None of the men had a history of gallstones or gallbladder disease.

After 14 years of follow-up, researchers found men who ate the most unsaturated fat were 18% less likely to develop gallstones compared with the men who ate the least.

Although this was an observational study, and researchers can't prove that the diets high in unsaturated fat were the only thing responsible for the reduction in gallstone risk, they say the findings support the already well-studied notion that eating a diet rich in unsaturated fats may provide a wealth of health benefits.

Constipation

Anyone who has eaten a "typical American, British, or Canadian diet" is very familiar with the symptoms of constipation. This is usually caused because of the low fiber content in the typical Western diet.

It results in decreased peristalsis, (muscular movement of the intestines) and decreased excretion of appropriate gastric and pancreatic enzymes, and consequently, constipation.

The chronic use of over the counter laxatives is very harmful to the body as it can paralyze the natural reaction to having peristalsis and normal functioning of the gastrointestinal tract. The occasional use of bowel stimulants – laxatives is all right if it is not used on a regular basis.

Both allopathic and herbal medicine offers various laxatives. Allopathic medicine utilizes various medications; some irritate the bowel, and some change the motility of the gut forcing fluid to enter the gut, and therefore, cause stool to move through faster. Most herbal preparations use anthraquinone laxatives based on senna and cascara.

Cholagogues stimulate the action of the liver and gallbladder with increased bile production, which stimulates peristalsis. The traditional herbs that are used in this type of stimulant include Barberry (berberis bulgaris), which is a bitter, cholagogue, and a hepatic stimulant.

Dandelion is a bitter glycoside, which exerts an astringent and antiseptic action on the gastrointestinal tract. Chelidonium Majus (Greater Celandine) is an herb containing various alkaloids that stimulate intestinal peristalsis and salivary secretions.

Certain essential oil fragments such as those containing ascaridole X and cymol have an antiseptic and cholinergic action on the gallbladder.

Tannins, which are contained, in tea extracts, exert an astringent effect on the gastrointestinal tract. They are helpful in patients who have utilized laxatives over a long period of time, and whose gastrointestinal tracts do not respond appropriately to normal diets.

The best way to avoid constipation is to make sure you have a significant amount of fiber in your diet. This does NOT mean taking a commercial fiber cereal in the morning. Although these do have some fiber, the good effect of these is offset by their high sugar or fat content.

A true high fiber cereal is not going to taste gourmet unless it is combined with lots of dried fruit, or other substances that will mollify the taste of the fiber. Fiber is bulk – that is why it works.

Fiber in your diet CAN be tasty if you consciously add lots of veggies, fruits (including but not limited to prunes) and whole grains. But if you cannot see fit to add it that way, try the following formula, the contents of which can be purchased in most bulk or health food stores:

Buy an equal quantity of the following 5 ingredients:

- ☑ Rice/or wheat bran
- ☑ Oat bran
- ☑ Psyllium husks
- ☑ Flax seed (light or dark)
- ☑ Spelt Bran

Make up a container with approximate equal quantities of each, mix well and then place 5 tablespoons of the mixture in boiling water. Add dried fruit and let sit until it congeals into a Jell-O-like substance. Put it in the fridge overnight and eat with yoghurt or just on its own. (If desired, this mixture can be consumed rapidly by filling a glass with water and drinking the combo until it is all gone from the bottom of the glass – at least 6 glasses of water, and not at a time you are taking any vitamins or medicines (the fiber can decrease their absorption).

The above is for the average person. As we age, we need more fiber, so just add a few more tablespoons, since it is low cal and all good for you anyway. You can also add other types of fiber and vary the combo with rye husks, soy husks, etc.

ADHD Attention Deficit Hyperactivity Disorder

ADHD or Attention Deficit Hyperactivity Disorder, also called ADD, refers to several problem behaviors all of which are associated with a poor attention span. This applies to children and adults.

ADHD children and adults are impulsive and disruptive interfering with learning and socializing. In adults, it can become less obvious but abnormal social behavior, addiction to drugs, and dependence on prescribed medication given over the years for presumed other diagnoses are common. It is believed that the cause of ADHD is biological, as well as environmental stressors. In recent years, research indicates that an ADHD food connection may also exist.

There has always been a speculation that food may play a role in ADHD. And although it may not be the only factor, studies also show that if certain foods and additives are eliminated, there can be a reduction in symptoms.

If you want to see if an ADHD food connection is responsible for some of an individual's behavior, eliminate the following foods from their diet for two weeks.

1. **No Dairy** – Cow's milk is the most important dairy product to eliminate so you should replace it with Almond, Soy, or Rice Milk. Since the brain is made up of 80% water, you should increase water intake.

2. **No Yellow Food** – Corn and squash are two yellow foods that need to be eliminated if there is an ADHD food connection. Bananas aren't yellow, just the skin is.

3. **No Junk Food** – Not sure what's junk food? If it comes out of a cellophane wrapper or the place you bought it has a big yellow arch outside, it's junk food, and could cause an ADHD food connection.

4. **No Fruit Juice** – When it comes to fruit juice, the bad outweighs the good, because of the high sugar content. One glass of apple juice contains the same amount of sugar as eight apples. Eat the apple, not the juice.

5. **Eliminate all other Sugar** – Sugar is the enemy and the cause of many health problems including an ADHD food connection.

6. **Eliminate Chocolate** – There should be no more than one piece of chocolate per week and that should be dark chocolate only.

7. **No NutraSweet or Splenda** – It's a common misconception that replacing sugar with NutraSweet or Splenda is good when, in fact, it's extremely bad for you. Stevia is from a root and does not cause problems and contains no chemicals or sugar so can be used to sweeten anything.

8. **No MSG** – It's a common ingredient in many foods –– not just Chinese food. It is used to enhance flavor, and it is responsible for many conditions. Processed meats are high in MSG, so they need to be avoided.

9. **No Food Coloring** – Reds and yellows are common colors related to ADHD food connection. Try to avoid all dyes if possible.

10. **No Meat** – Studies have shown that animal protein, particularly red meat (beef, pork, etc.) even if it is 'organic' and without all the antibiotics and hormones most commercially produced meat contains, aggravates ADHD and should be avoided.

The best way to avoid the ADHD food connection issues is to eat those natural foods that Mother Nature provides. When shopping for natural foods if you shop the outer aisles of the grocery store you are most likely to find "safe" foods. This is where the fresh fruit, vegetables, soy products, yoghurt, whole grain breads, fish, etc are usually located in many stores.

Alzheimer's Disease

There are many types of dementia where the brain does not keep up with the body in functioning. Alzheimer's disease (AD) is the most common dementia resulting in cognitive decline in people over the age of 65. It affects at least 4 million people in the USA, and it is the 4th leading cause of death. It costs society over $100 billion per year.

We do not know for sure what causes Alzheimer's, but there are many theories, and much research is being done to determine the etiology of this devastating disease. We know that it can affect people as early as 30 years of age, but this is a rare rapidly progressing form of the disease. More commonly, the disease affects those over the age of 65.

Because of the destruction of the nerve cells that control memory, thinking, and behavior the natural history of the disease progresses relatively predictably. The hippocampus and amygdala of the brain are affected at an early stage, leading to short-term memory loss and inability to do familiar tasks.

Later the cerebral cortex is affected which leads to alterations in language, reasoning, judgment, and behavior. Pathological changes are seen, with a high presence of amyloidal plaques, and neurofibrillary tangles. In most individuals, from onset to death, the disease usually takes about 8-10 years to manifest.

How to Diagnose Alzheimer's Disease

There is no perfect method as yet. Physicians and psychologists have developed various written tests and psychological testing devices that make one suspect the disease at an early stage. Once it has become evident, these tests can monitor the progress well.

Accurate observation, by the physician and a reliable observant/family member of the common symptoms, along with a physical examination, are the best method of diagnosis. In making the diagnosis, it is important to rule out potentially treatable diseases and conditions that can mimic AD.

If the onset of symptoms like focal neurologic findings, uncoordinated gait disturbances, or seizures is sudden in nature, it is unlikely that it is AD. Similarly in trying to diagnose AD, one must also rule out diseases such as brain tumors, chronic meningitis, subdural hematomas, chronic obstructive pulmonary disease (COPD), drug toxicity, electrolyte imbalances, psychiatric conditions, drug & alcohol abuse, endocrine disorders, and certain infections.

Early changes one often sees in a patient are generalized memory impairment; personality changes such as apathy, irritability, depression, anxiety; short-term memory loss; deterioration in judgment and social behavior, etc.

So if the police call you to inform you that your mother is wandering around your childhood home that was abandoned 40 years ago, she may be going through middle disease changes. Similar changes could be a decline in speech, verbal skills, and math skills; physical and verbal agitation in response to frustration; visual spacial dysfunction; paranoia, disorientation, etc.

While working on one cruise ship a, I remember a 90-year-old passenger in one of the suite cabins who came to the medical center wanting to get his INR checked to see if his blood was too thin, as his doctor back home had suggested. The test came back within the expected limits and I informed him of the same. He then told me that he had recently had a physical and that he was as healthy as a 30-year-old except for his eyesight. I thanked him for telling me that, but reminded him that he was on the blood thinner because of a history of atrial fibrillation and he should not try any really strenuous outings. He said he was okay with dying if he fell off a cliff or died in a scuba dive because he was not only at peace with God but that "God and I are tight. He knows I have poor eyesight, so he's fixed it so when I get up in the middle of the night to go to the bathroom, poof -- the light goes on. When I'm done, poof -- the light goes off and God had even accommodated him doing this in the suite just as he did at his home back in Georgia."

Based upon this discussion, since we had just had to disembark one passenger who was running down the halls trying to catch blue butterflies to the local psychiatric unit, I called his wife before he returned to his cabin to ask her if she had noticed any changes in his behavior. I mentioned to her his statement about his relationship with God and that he stated that he gets up during the night and "poof -- the light goes on in the bathroom and when he's done, poof -- the light goes off?"

"Oh my God!" his wife exclaimed. "He's peeing in the fridge, just like he does at home!"

Advanced changes include symptoms such as deterioration of bladder and bowel control, decline of the ability to speak and follow simple instructions, emotional disturbances, hallucinations, delusions, shuffling gait, slow and awkward movements, etc.

Finally, there are terminal changes, such as the inability to think, speak, perceive or move, etc.

When one has ruled out other potential causes of these conditions, then one can make the diagnosis of Alzheimer's. In short, this is not an easy disease to diagnose because it does mimic many others.

AD diagnosis is usually made by a clinical diagnosis. Laboratory tests are performed to identify treatable conditions. Accepted testing includes CBC, general chemistry test, thyroid test (severe hypo or hyper thyroidism), VDRL (tertiary or end stage syphilis), and B12 levels. CT and MRI's and other scanning testing are also done particularly if there is a rapid progression of symptoms, a suggestion of a vascular etiology, tumor or focal neurological signs. Genetic testing or DNA typing is also possible.

Therefore, by doing a physical examination, a neurological exam, a screening mental status exam, an interview of the patient, and a reliable caregiver and ruling out other treatable diseases, one can usually make the diagnosis of AD. Monitoring the progression of the disease, and then reevaluating every 6 months, or sooner, if deemed appropriate, is suggested.

Liver Disease

The liver is an extremely important organ in the human body. Metabolically the liver regulates a number of body functions. For example, it regulates the blood sugar level by storing sugar in the form of glycogen and releasing it gradually as required. The liver is also a "garbage processing factory" acting to eliminate a vast amount of body waste. When excess protein is consumed, it is converted by the liver to bile, which emulsifies it for urea and then eliminates it in the urine.

The liver is also a major storage center for Vitamins A, B12, D, E and K. The liver produces kupffer, which is important in the body's immune system. It also produces anti coagulants, which prevent clotting of the blood.

In its garbage processing function, (detoxification) the liver removes toxic substances produced by the body's metabolism in processing our food, and also various chemicals from the environment.

It removes these toxic substances from the blood and renders them less toxic and more water-soluble so that they can be filtered out by the kidneys, or excreted in the bile.

High fat and high protein diets (Atkins Diet, etc) make the liver work harder to detoxify these substances. The higher the protein content in the diet the higher the amount of toxic nitrogenous by-products made, which the liver has to break down.

In addition to these metabolically based stresses on the liver, excessive alcohol, and infections of the liver (hepatitis, etc), can also damage the cellular structure, making it more difficult for the liver to function normally and eliminate various metabolic toxins.

Hepatitis, which is inflammation of the liver, is usually caused by a variety of viruses: Hepatitis A, B, C, D, and E. Unfortunately they are very common viruses throughout the world creating significant pathology. We have effective vaccines for Hepatitis A & B available globally.

Yellow fever virus and cytomegalo viruses also cause liver problems, as do many others. In addition, to viral infections various bacteria can cause abscesses and other bacterial infections in the liver.

Certain parasites single out the liver for making themselves homes in which to multiply, and besides damaging the liver tissue itself, can create large abscesses that can cause a great deal of liver damage. An example of the latter is a protozoan called amoeba. Water-born protozoa are commonly found in many water supplies.

In addition to high protein, a high fatty diet or a diet high in alcohol, can result in cirrhosis of the liver where normal tissue is replaced by scar tissue. This scar tissue is obviously non-functional and consequently the liver fails to detoxify normal metabolic byproducts, putting the person is at risk for many potentially fatal conditions.

Treatments for Liver Disease

Unfortunately, short of a liver transplant, there is no treatment for end stage cirrhosis of the liver. There is also no known cure for most forms of viral hepatitis. However, there is some evidence showing partial reversal of symptomatology with a substance called interferon, but no cure.

Consequently, the best treatment we have available is to assist the body in healing itself, and hope that the damage that has been done is not too severe. An integral part of this recovery is avoidance of fatty foods, excess animal protein, alcohol, and environmental chemicals that can injure the liver.

Regular bowel movements, assisted by a high fiber diet are also important at helping the elimination of any of the toxic substances. A program of proper diet, extensive fluids, massage, therapeutic baths, and exercise is all part of a liver restoration program.

Certain herbs and foods will provide nutrients and help treat the liver. Licorice root is useful in regeneration; dandelion, skullcap and milk thistle are all known to help the liver. Double blind studies with an extract from milk thistle containing silymarin (sliybin) have shown favorable results in treating liver disease.

✓ Sulfur containing amino acids help prevent the accumulation of fat globules in the liver.

✓ Echinacea, Golden Seal, and Wild Indigo are known to stimulate the kupffer cells in the liver, if used in short term treatment.

✓ Vitamins A, B. C, and the mineral zinc are known to support the liver.

✓ Citric fruit juices and beets or beet juice are also beneficial to the liver.

✓ Foods such as artichoke and cucumber are traditionally known to help liver function.

✓ Garlic has an adjunctive use in treatment of Liver disease.

In many healing traditions, treatments have been developed to stimulate elimination of waste from the liver and increase bile flow.

In Southern India, there are traditional herbs that are said to open and cool the liver.

The American Native Indian tradition has herbs that are said to purify the blood and the lymph thereby purifying the liver. An example, of one of these liver-purifying treatments is:

• One cup of fresh squeezed orange juice with two tablespoons of lime or lemon juice. One cup of fresh water, ten drops of concentrated garlic oil, and one tablespoon of concentrated, fresh ginger juice.

• One tablespoon of olive oil – This should be blended or shaken well and drunk immediately.

• This is followed by two cups of dandelion tea and then no liquid or food for one hour. Then one should eat a bland carbohydrate food as the first meal (brown rice, potato, oatmeal, etc.). During a one-month treatment, you should take it for twelve days, stop for five, and then take it for another twelve days. If you follow this type of treatment it should be done for one month, twice a year.

Allergies

Common spring and summer allergies occur when your body reacts to certain molecules that exist in the environment. These molecules are called allergens.

These allergens are things that are common in the environment including dust, pollen, mold, etc. Although many people have allergies, these are things that most people do not react to. However, when your body overreacts to allergens, it causes symptoms like a runny nose, sneezing, watery eyes, etc.

Scientists believe that some people are born with allergies to certain allergens. You can also develop allergies later in your life, even to things that you were not previously allergic to.

It is not necessarily true that if you move away from a certain area, that you will never have allergies again. You can develop reactions to those allergens, or new ones, in the new area. (Sorry no medical validation for a move to Hawaii.)

In the spring the blooming of many plants begins. These plants shed pollen molecules, (allergens) which some people's bodies do not like. People often talk about hay fever. This is when you react to pollen allergens in the air.

The allergens that may affect you often depends on the climatic zone in which you are living. Remember, in the Southern Hemisphere the seasons are reversed with spring beginning in September, summer in December, fall in March, and winter in June.

If you are living in a temperate climate, like in the USA during late April and May, you can expect allergens due to tree pollen to be in the air and potentially causing you allergic symptoms. Allergies that occur late May to mid-July are often due to grass pollen, and those that occur late August until the frosts are often due to ragweed.

These are typical dates and change if you live in North Dakota vs. South Carolina, where the plants 'come alive' earlier. There are other allergens besides pollen that can cause spring - summer allergy type symptoms:

- **Mold** is a common allergen. It is most common where water collects, such as window moldings, basements with poor drainage, shower curtains, and in your garden around rotting logs, compost bins, leaf litter, and ornamental ponds. Mold allergies are common in places where the humidity is high in the summer or anytime where there is a lot of rainy weather (Vancouver!).

- **Pet Allergies** – People who are allergic to other animals are allergic to the allergens in the skin, hair, saliva, and urine of furry animals (pet dander). Hamsters, cats, and dogs are usually found guilty of this when you are both in a house where the animal lives and sheds some of its protein allergens.

- **Dust** – This can be either an allergen or an irritant. If it is "dirt dust" that bothers you, it is probably not a true allergy but rather sensitivity to the irritation of the dirt getting into your respiratory tract. If it is the tiny living creatures called dust mites that are causing the symptoms, then it is probably a true allergy. Dust mites live in bedding, carpets, mattresses, etc. and live on dead skin that is in the dust.

Common Allergy Symptoms:

- Stuffy nose
- Runny nose
- Sneezing
- Watery eyes
- Itchy eyes
- Itchy mouth
- Sinus pressure
- Ear pressure
- Hives
- Skin rashes
- Dark circles under the eyes

What You Can Do

There are things to do about allergies–you do <u>not</u> have to suffer.

1. Avoid the Allergens

- **Pollen** – Stay inside on dry, windy days. Keep doors and windows closed at home and in the car. Use an air conditioner with a good filter (i.e. HEPPA). Shower off the pollen on your skin/hair when you get home.

- **Pet Dander** – Vacuum regularly, brush and bathe pets often. If tests show you are allergic to that specific pet, you may have to find a new home for your pet. Don't be too quick to give Fido to Aunt Bessie, because pet dander mixes with house dust and can take a month or more to die down, so Fido may need a 2–3 month vacation at Bessie's house to determine if he is the cause.

- **Dust & Mites** – Wash bedding in water hotter than 130 degrees Fahrenheit every 7 days. Cover mattresses and pillows with plastic or special fabric covers. Mop the floor and wipe surfaces often with a damp cloth or one of the synthetic fiber dust mops.

  Vacuum everything regularly. Use an air cleaner with a particulate, HEPA, or electrostatic filter. Remove drapes, feather pillows, soft toys, & comforters until such time as you can determine that these mites are the offenders. Change carpets to wood, or tile floors or wash carpets with cleaners containing benzyl benzoate or tannic acid.

2. Boost Your Immune System

- Making your whole body healthier will reduce the likelihood that you will become sensitive to the allergens in the first place. If you have the allergies, boosting the immune system with plenty of sleep, nutritious food, regular exercise and antioxidants may help keep the symptoms shorter and/or less intense.

- Cutting out highly processed, high fat, high sugar foods from your diet will allow the body to fight off the allergens more effectively. Eat a high fiber diet with lots of fruit (Vitamin C) and leafy green vegetables.

- It is also very important to drink lots of fluids. If you allow the body to become dehydrated, then it can become more sensitive to a variety of potential invaders and irritants, like the allergens.

During allergy season, drink more than the recommended 8 glasses of water a day. If you live or work in an air-conditioned environment, then you should drink at least 3 liters of water in a 24-hour period. This not only makes sure you are well hydrated, but also flushes the system from the inside, of potential toxins. You will need to find where the restrooms are! Besides flushing the system, flush the tissues that are in first contact with the potential allergens–the nose/sinuses. Use a commercial saline rinse, or just use a Netty Pot/spray bottle with clean water and a pinch of salt. Spray or drain this fluid thru the nose/sinuses hourly while awake. It will take a while to get used to this, but you will get used to feeling better with this process.

3. Take Medication

- **Antihistamines**: If you take them before symptoms occur, they usually decrease a runny nose, sneezing, and itching. In other words, you take them as a preventative during the season. Some of the newer antihistamines such as Allegra or Zyrtec do not cause drowsiness.
  If you dislike taking pills, but find it hard to sleep at night due to your symptoms, use one of the older type antihistamines like diphenhydramine (Benadryl) before you go to bed. Using these will stop the symptoms and make you sleepy at the same time. The good night's sleep will help the body.

- **Pseudoephedrine**: It will temporarily decongest and relieve your stuffy nose, red eyes, etc. This class of medicine should not be taken for more than 3 days, or you can become addicted to it and feel worse when you stop using them. Pills, sprays, and drops are available over the counter.

- **Eye Drops**: Prescription steroids can be given by your doctor, but again should only be used for a short period of time. Avoid the Visine type over the counter meds for the eyes as they can addict your body so that if you do not use them, your eyes will run excessively.

- **Nasal Steroid Sprays**: Your doctor may prescribe this to reduce the reaction of the nasal tissues to inhaled allergens. These take a while to take effect but are better than the over the counter meds for your body.

- **Cromolyn Sodium Nasal Spray**: It helps prevent your body from reacting to the allergens. To be effective it must be started 3–4 weeks before the allergy season begins.

- **Allergy Shots**: Contain minute amounts of the allergen you are reacting to. Your family doctor or an allergist will determine what goes into these shots through skin allergy or blood testing. These shots are given on a regular basis (sometimes for years) so that your body gets used to the allergen and does not react with the usual symptoms.

The best approach is to get healthy, and keep your body healthy, and stay away from the allergens that you know you are allergic to.

Motion Sickness

Motion sickness is not just a problem for the sick, the elderly, or those of us that think of ourselves as wimps. Recent studies have reported that of 79 Space Shuttle (USA) missions, 94% of astronauts used some medication during flight. 47% of that medication was for the relief of space motion sickness.

If you suffer from seasickness, it can be rather annoying watching those that aren't affected going about their merry way, ever so happy and content, under the same conditions that have reduced you to complete misery.

Many first time passengers, on a variety of ships and boats, will be anxious about the possibility of seasickness, and the potential it has for disrupting their vacation. That anxiety, in and of itself, can have terrible effects.

How to Get Rid of Motion Sickness

If you suffer from true motion sickness due to an irritation of your middle ear, here are some suggestions that can help.

- ✓ **Pick the Right Seat** – If possible, sit in an area where you will receive the smoothest ride so you will feel less motion.

- When making a plane reservation, ask for a seat over a wing.
- Sit in the front seat of a vehicle.
- Sit near the front on a train.
- Book a cabin in the middle of a ship as far down as possible.

✓ **Avoid Standing** – The last thing you need when you are trying to keep your stomach happy is to be standing and get bounced around.

✓ **Face Front** – Never face backwards. Choose a seat that faces in the direction you are traveling so the body sees and feels the same thing.

✓ **Minimize Head Movements** – Try to avoid sudden movements of your head, which can make motion sickness worse.

✓ **Stay Outside** – When on a boat, you may be tempted to go below when you're feeling queasy. However, staying on deck is much better. That way your eyes can confirm the movement that your body is feeling.

✓ **Look Off Into the Distance** – Focus on a steady point away from the rocky boat, plane, or car. If there's no item, then stare out at the horizon, where the sky meets the earth (or water). This lets your eyes see that you are moving; matching the movement your body is feeling.

✓ **Leave Your Reading at Home** – When you read in a car, your eyes stay fixed on a stationery object, while your body feels the car's motion resulting in a sensory contradiction. Instead, focus on the road or scenery, and leave your reading at home.

✓ **Eat a Little or Don't Eat at All** – Sometimes eating helps, sometimes it doesn't. Experiment to see what works for you. To settle your stomach, about an hour before you leave, eat some plain crackers, a piece of bread, or some toast. A bit of plain yoghurt may help too. Avoid heavy foods and foods with odors that can prompt motion sickness.

✓ **Try OTC Remedies** – Antihistamines, such as Dramamine, Bonine, Gravol, and Marezine, should be taken at least an hour before the trip for maximum effectiveness.

✓ Always check the label for warnings and possible side effects, such as drowsiness or blurred vision, and take necessary precautions, such as not driving a car.

✓ **Motion Bands** – These are cloth bands with two plastic or metal pieces that push on your wrist, if placed properly on your wrist's (bottom) surface. Essentially, you are affecting the acupuncture points that may control the nausea. This works for some people.

✓ **Acidophilus Capsules** – The active ingredient in yogurt and other active intestinal bacteria can calm the stomach intestinal tract, when combined with tablets of Biotin (a B vitamin) can reduce motion sickness. Again, best to take before exposing the body to the excessive motion.

✓ **Keep Your Mind active** – Play mind games with the scenery, have heated discussions with fellow travelers, have someone read you a story, etc, but keep the mind active and off the motion.

Tattoos and Piercing Infection Risks

In some cultures, it is imperative that one has the proper number of tattoos. This is often a sign of tribal identification and progression through various stages of life.

In various African, South East Asian, and Polynesian cultures, lack of a tattoo can mean extrication from the usual society. Add to this the piercing of various portions of the body, and one has the needed cultural accoutrements of certain tribal societies.

Piercings can entail objects placed, in ever increasing sizes, thru a body part, so that eventually that body part is deformed in a way that is either considered beautiful or spiritual.

Examples of this include the use of weights and various objects, which are placed in the ear lobes, to increase their size. Some Buddhist sects value the elongated ear lobes, which can traditionally be seen in the scripture of that religion.

I remember one holiday celebration in southern India where various iron rods were pierced thru the cheeks of the mouth, and the participant was then given objects to pull with the iron bar-like a rail car. Some had hooks attached to their backs by which they pulled carts or autos. The above being a way of demonstrating their religious devotion.

Why am I bringing up the practice of tattooing and piercing in a book on health maintenance and improvement? No recommendations to partake! If one follows certain beliefs, one would not put anything in the ear that could interrupt the flow of energy (Chi).

From an infectious disease point of view, piercing provides an ideal portal for bacteria and viruses. One needs to meticulously maintain it from an antibacterial point of view.

Tattooing, on the other hand, provides the ideal entry into the body of viruses from contaminated needles. Innumerable examples of the spread of blood borne diseases (hepatitis B and HIV in particular) have been documented from Tattoo parlors worldwide. The dye used in the tattoos themselves is also suspect in cases of mercury & cadmium poisoning.

Not to sound too old or intolerant of new styles, I must also comment on my personal dislike of the disfigurement of otherwise very attractive young people of both sexes who have placed bars, pins, studs and the like thru every conceivable orifice and non-orifice.

I am still clinically surprised when examining an attractive young lady, conservatively and appropriately dressed for a visit to the doctor, who opens her mouth and reveals a metal stud (or plastic) in the middle of the tongue. The dental damage, speech impediment, and unexpected damage are evident.

One physical I was doing on a young female revealed 27 piercings and 14 tattoos. She had lips, eyebrows, nose, breasts, umbilicus, vulva, clitoris, earlobes, etc, pierced; and her male friend had similar piercings including the tip of his penis.

The nurse who accompanied me in the exams was even more shocked than I. The man's tattoo had an eagle across his chest (that flapped when he flexed his pectoral muscles) -- his nipple rings had little bells on them so that as the eagle flapped its wings, the bells tinkled. I won't mention what the penis piercing had. My nurse and I could hardly keep a straight face.

Mosquito Borne Disease

Mosquitoes - there was a time that these little creatures were little more than an annoyance. However, these days being bitten by a mosquito actually poses a serious health risk. In many parts of the world, malaria is carried by the mosquito and kills many innocent victims.

In North America, there is the worry of the West Nile Virus; it has become a summer threat across North America. The first case was diagnosed in 1999, and since then that little buzz sets fear into the recipient that hears it. Government agencies find themselves in a dilemma, because North Americans are either not taking the West Nile Virus seriously enough, or they are taking it far too seriously, living in fear.

The reality is that the West Nile Virus should not force you into spending the summer indoors, but you also need to be prepared to take precautions against mosquitoes and the West Nile Virus.

The risk of being infected with West Nile Virus is less than 1% -- so go ahead, enjoy your summer -- just take some precautions, and make sure your precautions aren't putting you at greater risk than the virus you are trying to avoid.

Mosquito Statistics

1 in 10 people are highly attractive to mosquitoes. We do know that genetics accounts for a whopping 85% of our susceptibility to mosquito bites. Certain elements of our body chemistry that, when found in excess on the skin's surface, make mosquitoes swarm closer.

People with high concentrations of steroids or cholesterol near the skin surface attract mosquitoes. Mosquitoes also target people who produce excess amounts of certain acids, such as uric acid (gout). Any type of carbon dioxide is attractive, even over a long distance to the mosquitoes.

Obese people tend to give off more carbon dioxide, than thin ones, which is why mosquitoes typically prefer munching on adults rather than small children. Movement and heat also attract mosquitoes.

Even if your body chemistry doesn't attract mosquitoes, where you're located might. While any water source is potential breeding grounds for mosquitoes, they much prefer stagnant water. Mosquitoes have been around for 170 million years -- and there are more than 175 known species in the U.S alone and more overseas.

Ways to Keep Mosquitoes Away

Chemical Mosquito Repellent

The majority of available mosquito repellants derive their effectiveness from chemicals. Protecting the public from mosquitoes since 1957, DEET continues to be the chemical of choice used in repellants. In repeated studies, it's been proven the most effective chemical repellant on the market.

Repellants with 23.8% DEET (most formulas contain between 10% and 30%) protect wearers for about five hours. DEET has been in use for over 40 years and has a remarkable safety record. Only a few hospitalizations have been reported, mainly due to gross overuse.

Avoid Health Problems When Using DEET:

- ✓ Follow label directions and precautions.
- ✓ Use sparingly.
- ✓ Avoid spraying on or near cut skin, eyes, mouth, and nose, under clothing, or near food.
- ✓ Wash treated skin with soap and water when you go indoors.
- ✓ Spray on clothes or pre-treat clothes and only use on exposed areas of skin.

Precautions for use on children:

Select the lowest concentration effective for the amount of time spent outdoors. Avoid use on infants less than 2 months of age. Avoid repeated applications, which may increase the potential toxic effects of DEET.

Non-Chemical Mosquito Repellant

For those of you who hate chemical sprays, there are some alternatives. Let's look at some of those alternatives.

Skin So Soft

Apply Avon Skin so Soft, a non-toxic oil based spray that works until it evaporates, so it needs to be reapplied every 12 to 15 minutes.

Soybean Repellant

A soybean oil-based repellant is able to protect you from mosquito bites for about 1.5 hours.

Natural Oils

- Researchers found other oils -- citronella, cedar, peppermint, lemongrass, and geranium -- provide short-lived protection at best. Oil-of-eucalyptus products may offer longer-lasting protection.

- Citronella candles, incense and coils, can keep most mosquitoes at bay, but they will not keep the stubborn ones from sneaking through and biting.

Oil of Lemon Eucalyptus

- ✓ Approved by the US Centers for Disease Prevention and Control.

- ✓ Oil of lemon eucalyptus is natural, plant-based repellent oil that is prepared from leaves of Eucalyptus citronella.

✓ Oil of lemon eucalyptus is said to be is similar in effect to a low-concentration of mosquito repellant with DEET.

✓ It is also known as p-methane 3, 8-diol or PMD.

Mosquito Netting

✓ Mosquito netting has long been used in tropical countries and is seen more often in North America since the West Nile Virus migrated to North America in 1999.

✓ Mesh with holes 1.2 mm x 1.2 mm is recommended.

✓ Mosquito netting is available in tarps, infant netting, hanging erect tents, in mosquito head nets and full body nets for between $5 and $100 online.

✓ Now, U.S. and Canadian citizens living in mosquito infested areas, near standing water, or when traveling to cottage country in damp summer months, should wear mosquito netting for protection against mosquitoes, black flies and other biting insects.

✓ For the best protection, mosquito netting should have mesh large enough for air circulation, but small enough to keep out mosquitoes.

✓ When working or walking in mosquito-populated areas polyester or polyamide mosquito netting is best because it offers lightweight, long-lasting protection, and is available in various mesh sizes.

✓ Mosquito netting made of cotton, is more susceptible to dampness, and weighs more. However, when sleeping outdoors, cotton mosquito netting is considered to offer the best sleeping comfort, and it can be sprinkled with water to keep cool, and promote air circulation. It can also be sprayed with various mosquito repellents.

Carbon Dioxide Devices

- The carbon dioxide device is also called the mosquito magnet.

- It is said to emit carbon dioxide, which will attract the mosquitoes.

- There have been no studies to support this claim. However, the US Coast Guard does comment that they are effective mosquito traps.

Electronic Devices

- Electronic bug zappers attract insects to the ultraviolet light and then send a lethal electrical charge that fries the bugs.

- Bug zappers can lure and kill more than 10,000 insects in a single evening. They do not discriminate between insects, but they tend to kill the insects that are attracted to ultraviolet light, which mosquitoes are <u>not</u>.

- However, studies show that 90% of what bug zappers fry are non-biting insects – including insects that might eat pesky mosquitoes, such as dragonflies.

- Mosquitoes prefer human targets to ultraviolet light, so bug zappers usually catch only 3% of the mosquitoes in your yard, if that.

- Ultrasonic mosquito devices are said to repel mosquitoes by emitting a high pitch noise that is supposed to sound like their natural predator, the dragonfly. It doesn't work on deaf mosquitoes.

Vitamin B

Research has shown if you take <u>large</u> quantities of Vitamin B that the mosquitoes will run the other way. You have to take enough of it to allow your skin to smell of Vitamin B, so the amount in a multivitamin is not enough. You can get a B vitamin complex at your local mall. Try taking 2 or so a day (100mg tabs) and keep increasing the dose until you can smell it on your skin. At worst, it will help deal with stress and keep away the people you don't like anyway.

Clothing

Long sleeved shirts and pants will also help somewhat but are no guarantee. Obviously heavier material will give the best protection. You can spray your clothes with pyrethrin, let dry, and the mosquitoes will not bite through the cloth. It acts as a repellent also.

Scents

Probably most important is not wearing any perfume or any other scented lotions or sprays. This attracts mosquitoes and black flies like crazy!

Bounce

US Postal service sent out a message to all letter carriers to put a sheet of Bounce in their uniform pockets to keep yellow jackets away. They also keep mosquitoes away. This means they are great for sports in the evening. Tie a Bounce sheet through your belt loop to repel mosquitoes.

Travel Vaccinations

Depending on where you are headed, you may need certain vaccinations to enter and leave the country and should take others anyway. How do you find out which ones you need, how far in advance you need to get them, and where you can get them? Websites from the US & British (NHS) governments and the World Health Organization (WHO) will give the information needed.

Generally speaking, you probably won't need many vaccinations other than an update on your basic ones, unless you are going to Asia, South Asia, Africa or South America.

If you are going to one of these continents, it's best to do a little homework in advance of your trip. Remember that many vaccinations take several days to months to begin protecting you, so start planning as soon as you book your flight.

A good resource for getting started is the Center for Disease Control's Travel Information (CDC) site. Besides the routine information, the site has information on children, adults, and those with compromised immune systems. The site also places special focus on yellow fever vaccination. This is because it is the vaccination most often required by travelers entering endemic countries.

Check this site for rules regarding your exact travel itinerary. You might be allowed to enter Brazil and Senegal from the U.S. for example, but if your travel plans include a flight directly from Brazil to Senegal, you will need to make sure your vaccinations are still valid. Check this site and others to determine if you need prophylaxis for malaria or need to be cautious about other insect borne diseases.

Immunizations are recorded on your International Certificate of Vaccination, the yellow health card. Your doctor has the authority to fill this out for some vaccinations. But the Yellow Fever & Cholera vaccines must be given and stamped by a county health department official, or a Travel Medicine Clinic that has obtained permission to stamp certificates. Carry this International Certificate of Vaccination with you on your trip.

Most importantly, if you are pregnant, have an immunodeficiency or are traveling with a child, please consult your doctor about immunizations. Many vaccinations are considered unsafe for these travelers, and all care must be taken to protect your health.
If you cannot receive a vaccination for any valid reason, make sure to carry a certificate from your health care provider verifying your condition.

Recommended sources/links include:

Centers for Disease Control and Prevention
(CDC) – http://www.cdc.gov
Department of Health
http://www.dh.gov.uk
Foreign & Commonwealth Office
http://www.fco.gov.uk
Health Protection Agency UK
http://www.hpa.org.uk (malaria)
Health Protection Scotland

http://www.hps.scot.nhs.uk/
Joint Committee on Vaccination and Immunization
http://www.advisorybodies.doh.gov.uk/jcvi/fol_classesofinformation.htm
National Travel Health Network and Centre (NaTHNaC)
http://www.nathnac.org
World Health Organization (WHO)
http://www.who.int/en/
HO disease outbreak news
http://www.who.int/csr/don/en/
ISTM TravelMedListserve
https://www.istm.org
British Mountaineering Council
http://www.thebmc.co.uk/
Health Advice for Travelers
http://www.dh.gov.uk/PolicyAndGuidance/HealthAdviceForTravellers/fs/en
Fitfortravel
http://www.fitfortravel.scot.nhs.uk/
TRAVAX advice line
http://www.travax.scot.nhs.uk/
Promed
http://www.promedmail.org

Travel Tips – Staying Healthy

There is nothing worse than getting sick while you are on vacation. Getting hurt can be even worse. In order to get well as quickly as possible, here are some suggestions for getting through an unplanned illness or injury while traveling.

- Prevention is the best policy. Depending on how exotic your destination is you may be required to prove you've had certain vaccinations. Remember to bring the documentation with you.

- Look into traveler's insurance. Your home health insurance probably will not cover you abroad, so this insurance can save you a lot of money if you need a hospital or specialist. You can also purchase insurance that covers transporting you out of Timbuktu or similar place without appropriate medical care.

- These Air Evacuation services are sometimes attached to traditional Travel Insurance packages, but the more comprehensive ones are separate (and not very expensive) policies (SOS, MedjetAssist, Aeromed, AirMed Assist, AeroCare Air Ambulance, etc, etc)

- Pack all necessary medications in your carryon bag, in case your luggage is delayed or lost, and keep them in their original containers, in case of inspection at the airports. If your medications are unusual, you should bring a doctor's note with you to attest that you need it.

- It's always advisable to pack a small first aid kit. Although in many westernized countries you can find most of these basic items easily, the speed of having the appropriate item handy is helpful. If you are on the move a lot, in a Third World country, or don't trust your language skills, it can be helpful to have this kit with you.

- It should include bandages, anti-diarrhea medication such as Pepto Bismol, decongestant, insect repellent, sunscreen, a digital thermometer, and aspirin or other pain medication, calamine or antihistamine cream, and a sanitary hand wipes.

- Additionally, you may want to pack small scissors, tweezers, medical tape and gauze for emergencies, especially if you are traveling with children, who tend to be accident-prone when we least expect it! Pack it in the checked baggage.

Think about where you are going, and use your best judgment, as well as suggestions from guidebooks or tourism websites. Have a safe and enjoyable trip!

Heat Illness and Dehydration:

Protecting Yourselves

With the hot days of summer come summer sports like baseball, tennis, and football, played both in the neighborhood and at camp. Before you send the kids out to practice sports, or even just for a long day of play in the sun, you need to learn how to protect your child and yourself against the dangers of dehydration and heat illness.

What Puts Us at Risk for Dehydration?

- Prolonged exposure to high temperatures, direct sun, and high humidity, without sufficient rest and fluids.

- Older people have less heat tolerance due to their circulatory system, and a decreased skin resistance to the elements. A child's body surface area makes up a much greater proportion of his overall weight than an adult's, which means children face a much greater risk of dehydration and heat-related illness.

Signs of Dehydration

Early signs of dehydration include:

- Fatigue
- Lack of energy
- Thirst
- Dry lips and tongue
- Feeling overheated

If you wait to drink until you feel thirsty, you're already dehydrated. Thirst doesn't really kick in until you have lost 2% of body weight as sweat and loss through respiration

Untreated dehydration can lead to three more types of heat illness:

- ✓ Heat Cramps: Painful cramps of the abdominal muscles, arms, or legs.

- ✓ Heat Exhaustion: Dizziness, nausea, vomiting, headaches, weakness, muscle pain, and sometimes unconsciousness.

- ✓ Heat Stroke: A temperature of 104 or higher, and severe symptoms, including nausea and vomiting, seizures, disorientation or delirium, lack of sweating, shortness of breath, unconsciousness, and coma.

- Both heat exhaustion and heat stroke require immediate care. **Heat stroke is a medical emergency** that when untreated can be deadly.

How to Prevent Dehydration

☑ Make sure that you drink water and occasionally sports drinks, but be careful with these beverages as they often have way too much sugar in them, and some have lots of caffeine, so read the label!

☑ Drink fluids early and often. Before you go out to practice or play, make sure you are fully hydrated by drinking plenty of water, juice, etc.

☑ Then, during play, make sure you take regular breaks to drink fluid, even if you do not feel thirsty.

☑ Get acclimatized before summer practice to slowly build up your fitness and ability to handle the heat.

☑ Know that dehydration is cumulative. You can gradually develop a more severe dehydration over a few days and it won't show up right away.

☑ A simple rule of thumb: if your urine is dark in color, rather than clear, or light yellow, you may be becoming dehydrated.

Treating Heat Illness

The first thing you should do with any heat illness is get out of the sun into a cool, comfortable place and start drinking plenty of cool (not cold) fluids.

Take off any excess layers of clothing or bulky equipment. You can put cool, wet cloths on overheated skin. In cases of heat cramps, gentle stretches to the affected muscle should relieve the pain.

Heat stroke is <u>always an emergency</u> and <u>requires immediate medical attention.</u>

The Risk of Dehydration from Heat Illness

One of the biggest risk factors is a previous episode of dehydration or heat illness. Other factors that can put you at greater risk for heat illness include obesity, recent illness (especially vomiting or diarrhea), and use of antihistamines or diuretics.

Lack of acclimatization to hot weather, and exercising beyond your level of fitness can also lead to heat illness. If you are not in shape, and try to go out and do things quickly, or if you are not used to that kind of heat and humidity, and duration of exercise, that sets you up for dehydration and heat illness.

Don't Practice Sports When It's Too Hot

A growing number of athletic programs suggest that it is sometimes too hot to practice. In fact, many are restricting outdoor practice when the National Weather Service's heat index rises above a certain temperature. The heat index, measured in degrees Centigrade or Fahrenheit, is an accurate measure of how hot it really feels, when the relative humidity is added to the actual temperature.

In certain countries where the ambient temperature is excessive (Saudi Arabia, United Arab Emirates, etc,) sports facilities have been constructed to allow people to play in more moderate temperatures and avoid frequent trips to the hospital (they even have an indoor ski hill.)

Surgical Healing

Many people avoid ever having a second or third surgery. Some even avoid the first one because of the fear of not healing. Some people avoid surgeries, because they bleed abnormally, some because they have reactions to anesthesia, some fear being asleep, while still others fear the pain of any surgical procedure and its potential consequences. I have found in my clinical practice over the years that the main reason people shun surgery is the post surgical complications and discomfort that is common.

Cause of Surgical Problems

What causes post surgical problems and discomfort? In many instances, it is the nature of the procedure itself. If you are going to cut and slash a tissue that is not ready to be mutilated, it is going to bring forth any and all defenses it has in an effort to try and defend itself and repair what it can. The human body has some pretty elaborate defense systems.

Liposuction

As an example of an invasive procedure, let's look at the now popular plastic surgical procedure of liposuction. This cosmetic procedure removes extra fat cells from various portions of the body. In some instances, large portions of fat are removed from the abdomen or legs. In others, a very delicate removal is done from around the eyes or on the chin. In reality, it is a rather forceful insult to the body.

A cut is made in the area to liposuction, a tube is inserted, and in the space where the fat lies (subcutaneous tissue) a large quantity of water and local anesthetic are instilled. The calculation of this is important so as not to overburden the body with this fluid or with the anesthetic.

Once this fluid is in place, another tube is inserted and the fat cells are removed by suction in a sweeping motion, over and over. This also sucks up supporting tissues, small nerves, and blood and lymph vessels in the process.

There is another liposuction technique that involves the same basic technique (tumescent) described above with the addition of ultrasound. This is believed to break up the fat cells more, and facilitate the removal of the fat. According to statistics there tend to be more complications, especially burns, with this technique–and consequently more needed healing.

As one can readily see, with either technique, there is a lot of tissue trauma that obviously occurs with liposuction from the technical side. This results in massive bruising and collections of fluid–mostly lymphatic fluid. This is so significant that the standard post surgical technique for liposuction patients is to receive a body girdle of the portion of the body that has been suctioned, in an attempt to reduce the massive swelling.

This swelling is the body's method of defending itself. Massive amounts of trauma, and the body place large amounts of fluid between the traumatized areas and the skin to protect the raw areas. Makes perfect sense, but it is said to be terribly uncomfortable and painful from all the patients I have interviewed. If the swelling is too great, it can actually increase the time necessary to heal.

Continuing with the liposuction example, let's look at some other things that can be done to assist in promoting post surgical healing, and things that can be done in preparation for having any elective surgery done.

As mentioned above with liposuction and many surgical maneuvers, there is often swelling (edema) following the procedure. Making those tissues healthy before hand is the logical method of assisting the body.

Therapeutic Massage

Therapeutic massage, from a qualified therapist, is one of the first things that is helpful. Getting tissues that may have not been 'awake' for a long time ready to work is a simplified way of thinking of massage.

Massage before and after a surgical procedure, done in the proper manner, can stimulate lymphatic drainage and initiate the immune system to kick into action in working at repairing the damage that may have occurred post surgically. This is very obvious, when observing the massage techniques used in certain Eastern based therapeutic methodologies (Ayurveda, Thai massage, etc).

The very basis of the application of some medications in Ayurveda is with massage. It is believed that if the medicated oils are massaged into the body, they will have more beneficial effects than those same ingredients taken by mouth. In fact, in the tradition of Ayurveda, certain herbal preparations are only applied by massage. We discuss this method of various medical treatments in other parts of this book.

It is important to have a massage therapist who knows what they are doing, specifically in the post-surgical period. As any Certified Hand Therapist CHT (Physical/Occupational therapists who specialize in the treatment of the upper extremities) will tell you, it is critical that only the appropriate amount of stretching and tissue massage be carried out after most surgical procedures on the hand.

If too much stretching or pressure is applied, the result can be disastrous with lax ligaments a potential result. If insufficient stretching/massage occurs, contractures (areas where the tissues are too tight and cannot function properly) may result in a hand that does not work.

A deep tissue masseuse, bunter massage practitioner, or Rolfing practitioner who applies their technique post surgically with vigor can actually cause more tissue damage than doing nothing at all. One has to remember that there is damaged tissue under the surface skin, and it has to be gently handled.

If a therapist who has experience with this is unavailable, it is better to do the massage yourself or get a loved one to learn the techniques. Most public libraries and natural food stores have books on massage techniques.

Most large cities have massage schools. Use toning massage methods pre-surgically, and lymphatic drainage techniques post surgically. These are the most common massage techniques used. Specialized Ayurvedic massage techniques with specific therapeutic oils will address specific post surgical situations.

Post Op Herbs and Vitamins

Using various topically applied oils and herbal preparations can, in and of themselves, be beneficial pre and post surgically. The oil from the neem plant is well known throughout Asia to be therapeutically beneficial to healing skin.

Neem Oil

Neem is a healing herb. This is a plant found commonly in the Indian subcontinent. It is a major 'cure all' herb that is used in the medicine cabinets in India – from the poorest peasant to the president. For pre-surgical preparation, take 2 capsules of neem leaves three times a day a week before surgery. Neem oil can be used post surgically for wound healing. Caution it has a pungent odor.

Aloe Vera

Aloe Vera preparations can tone skin pre-surgically.

Vitamin E

Vitamin E oil may be helpful post surgically in reducing scar formation after the acute phase (i.e. after the sutures are removed). Vitamin E taken internally in large quantities pre surgically or immediately post surgically can actually increase bleeding and should be avoided in large quantities (over 800 IU).

Arnica

In the English Homeopathic tradition, the preparation called Arnica Montana is traditionally known to assist in pre-surgical preparation of tissues and to reduce swelling post surgically. It is used in the 5c, 6c, 30c, or 200X doses. The traditional recommendation for this medication is to dissolve one of the homeopathic pills under the tongue three times a day three days before surgery.

After surgery, the dose is increased to 3 pills three times a day for 5 days. Then for the following 7 days, one pill a day under the tongue. As with all homeopathic medications, they are not to be touched with the fingers. Once they are taken, one is not to eat or drink for 20-minutes. Homeopathic medications are described in other parts of the book. They are minute does of a substance that mimics the problem the person is having – a symptom imitator.

Vitamins

In the American vitamin supplement tradition, there are many vitamins that are said to assist in pre and post surgical situations.

Bromelain

Bromelain – 1500 mg three times a day between meals with water 5 days prior to surgery is said to help. This is to be continued for two weeks after surgery.

Zinc

Zinc is best taken prior to surgery. It reduces the time it takes for wounds to heal, quickly reduces wound size, and boosts the immune system to ward off infection. Zinc deficiency is common in the United

States, which is why many doctors recommend taking 30 mg of zinc orally a day, for 4 to 6 weeks, so that you have adequate zinc levels by surgery time. If you undergo surgery deficient in zinc, it will slow your recovery time.

Chlorella

Japanese studies have shown Chlorella Growth Factor (CGF) to be very effective in speeding up cell growth, which is a major factor in the natural repair and healing of wounds. When taken internally, it acts as an immune booster, and when applied topically, it functions as a protective cleansing compound for the skin, but makes it green.

Gotu Kola

For centuries Gotu Kola has been used as natural medicine in Asia. It helps in treating scars and wounds with infections that have not yet reached the bone. Gotu Kola when applied externally increases the level of antioxidants locally and helps to repair connective tissues.

Colloidal Silver

Colloidal Silver can be used topically to prevent infections. It works better than antibiotics and stops bacteria from having the opportunity to build up resistance. It stains the skin temporarily with a blackish color.

Astragalus

Astragalus contains a number of trace minerals, and micronutrients. This herb aids in support of the healing process.

Vitamin C

Vitamin C is an important component for full post-operative recovery. It has been shown that levels of this compound actually drop in burn victims, post-op patients, and other types of physical trauma. Vitamin C is required to make collagen, which is the connective tissue in the skin that helps healing to occur.

Self Massage

Massaging oneself pre-surgically with various aromatic oils, like lavender, added to walnut oil or almond oil can also be beneficial to the health of the skin and subcutaneous tissues. For someone who is not used to massaging themselves with oils, or creams on a regular basis, like most of the American male population, doing so can be considered either a chore or a new experience.

The post surgical result will be less positive for those who do not change the perception of self-massage from being a chore to being a therapy. An important therapeutic step in the healing process is to get to know your own body, and getting to accept it as it is.

It is also important that you get to know your body in a manner, where subtle changes will be noticed. When you know how your body feels, and how certain levels of pressure feel, any significant or subtle change reported to the doctor can catch problems before they become big problems.

Obviously, you can't massage all parts of your body unless you are a supreme contortionist. Knowing, or being able to do all the appropriate massage techniques post surgically is also impossible.

Having a therapist who works with you on a regular basis can be helpful, as it will allow them to note various changes as they occur. The therapist who has a good technique can be a beneficial assistant to the surgeon in monitoring the post surgical course.

Thus far, I have been speaking mostly of techniques that are beneficial to the skin and superficial tissues, for procedures like liposuction. These same therapeutic techniques can also aid surgical techniques that involve organs deep in the body. This applies to the superficial scars that are needed to close the wound after open-heart surgery, gall bladder surgery, bowel resection, etc.

Other Post Surgery Techniques

With appropriate massage (albeit very gently) the internal organs can be stimulated to begin to function again more rapidly after surgery. Techniques such as Reiki have also been shown to be effective in this manner.

Gentle exercise (like gentle swimming or walking in a pool) following bowel resection has been shown to restart the peristalsis (normal intrinsic motion of the bowels) faster than subjects that simply lay in bed.

Early mobilization after hip replacement surgery has shown that final outcomes are significantly better, than for those that 'take the bed rest' after the surgery. Most hospitals now start some form of physical therapy almost immediately after hip and knee replacement surgery.

In addition to the American herbal/vitamin tradition, for centuries, the Ayurvedic medical system and the Chinese medical system have had a variety of herbs in their armamentarium, that are specific for tissue healing (post operative) and tissue resilience (in preparation for surgery).

CHAPTER 6
CANCER PREVENTION

Because Cancer in its many forms has had the attention of researchers and practitioners for many years, the subject of cancer prevention has also caught their attention at many prestigious and famous medical centers throughout the world.

It has also involved the ingenuity of many charlatans, who prey on all individuals who do not want to hear the three most dreaded words in the English language 'You've got cancer.'

Fortunately, we are now able to diagnose the disease in its many forms much earlier than previously, and effect various treatments that are often able to arrest or cure the disease.

Unfortunately, many of the treatments are as bad or worse than the disease itself in the discomforts they create. And, as we well know, if you can prevent something it is always easier and more effective than having to treat the condition after you get it.

Cancer Statistics

Some statistics indicate that nearly one third of the American population will have some form of cancer in their lifetime. If we look at some of these statistics, it is certainly a disease that needs to be reckoned with:

- 2 million new cases of cancer are diagnosed in the USA every year.

- There are 500,000 annual deaths from cancer in the USA

- 11 million are still living with one of the one hundred different diseases that are classified as cancer.

- Cancer is an expensive disease. It costs many people their life savings and stretches some insurance companies into bankruptcy.
- The US government has invested $30 billion in cancer research in the last 30 years, and billions more have been raised from private sources to help understand and wipe out the disease.

- At least one half of all cancers can be linked to exposures to environmental factors such as the sun's UV rays, radiation, pesticides, air pollution, and smoking/second hand smoke.

- The other half of the overall risk of getting cancer can be attributed to one's diet.

Why Cancer Rates Vary From Country to Country

The total weight of evidence about a nutritional approach to the prevention of disease has reached a critical mass. M Gaynor MD (a NYC Oncologist) has gathered numerous medical studies that demonstrate the major influence of nutrition on cancer.

A hundred and fifty years ago, the odds of dying of cancer were 1/150 deaths. Today more than 500,000 deaths in America are due to cancer lowering the odds to 1/8 deaths.

Cancer rates vary dramatically between countries, none more so than between Japan and the USA. Overall age adjusted cancer rates in the USA are more than 50% higher than in Japan. Americans have a 30% chance of developing cancer and an 11.2% chance of dying from it by the age of 75, compared to a 20.4% chance of developing cancer and a 9.7% chance of dying from it in Japan.

The only common forms of cancer that are more prevalent in Japan are pancreatic, liver, colorectal, and stomach cancer. The following table shows age adjusted cancer rates per 100,000 people for both the United States and Japan.

Cancer Type	USA Rate	Japan Rate
Prostate	83.8	22.7
Lung	42.1	24.6
Breast	76	42.7
Colorectal	29.2	31.5
Melanoma	14.3	0.5
Non–Hodgkin lymphoma	13.7	5.1
Bladder	12.7	4.8
Kidney	12.1	4.9
Thyroid	9.9	3.1
Leukemia	9.9	4.3
Pancreatic	7.0	7.9
Liver	4.5	11.2
Stomach	5.7	31.1
Overall	335.0	201.1

The Cancer Prevention Food List

Although no one knows for sure, the most recent research indicates that the following foods are helpful in the potential prevention of cancer. This is NOT to say that all of these foods are good for everyone. They may actually be detrimental for some.

It is very important to determine with your doctor what is right for you and your particular condition. In other parts of this book, we will cover other foods and supplements that may also be helpful. Here goes with the list:

✓ All vegetables, but especially those in the cabbage family and root plants; Brussels sprouts, cabbage, cauliflower, kale, okra, turnips, yams, broccoli, potatoes, green beans, peas, carrots, etc.

✓ Most fruits, but especially citrus fruits like orange and grapefruit.

- ✓ Soy foods, this includes the many forms of tofu, tempeh, cooked soybeans, soy protein based meat substitutes
- ✓ Tomatoes, which are actually classified as a fruit
- ✓ Raw onions and garlic
- ✓ All whole grains like wheat, oats, barley, rye, brown rice, quinoa, millet
- ✓ Most nuts
- ✓ Some mushrooms (especially Shiitake, Reishi & Maitake)
- ✓ All legumes like red and green lentils
- ✓ Decaffeinated green tea
- ✓ Olive oil

For the most part, this is a list of fairly healthy foods in general. Throughout the book, you'll see mention of most of these cancer prevention foods because most of them are good for other aspects of your heath too. But remember, some are not good for certain conditions. For example, excessive amounts of tomatoes can aggravate arthritic conditions extensively.

Supplements for Preventing Cancer

Many researchers indicate that there are various supplements that can be helpful in preventing the disease. Some of these supplements have undergone controlled studies that show a decrease in abnormal cell growth (the basis of what cancer really is) when these supplements are taken on a regular basis.

Some people claim that these nutrients should all be available in a good balanced diet, and that there is no need for supplementation. This might be true if you include pine bark tea, and grape seeds in your regular diet, but most of us do not. We usually don't eat the quantities of these foods necessary to possibly prevent cancer.

Further, the soil that many of our foods is grown or grazed on is severely deficient of the essential nutrients needed to prevent cancers, etc. Furthermore, because of the omnipresent chemical fertilizers used to make crops 'bright and green' and economically feasible, many of the nutrients that are in the soil are chemically blocked by these fertilizers and plant enhancers.

In any event, the following is gleaned from a number of research papers, and health gurus as being appropriate as a daily regime. Make sure you balance this with a good multivitamin (see supplements section of book):

Selenium 200 mcg

Vitamin C 2,000 mg

L–lysine   2000 mg

Vitamin D 400 IU

Vitamin E 400 IU

Vitamin B complex 100mg (of each)

Mixed carotenoids 5,000 IU beta

carotene

Alpha carotene 1,000 IU

Lutein 6 mg

Lycopene 10 mg

Calcium 2,000 mg (much more needed for bones, etc)

Alpha–linolic acid 100mg

N–acetyl–cysteine 600mg

Folic acid 400 mcg

Magnesium 1000 mg

Grape seed extract 25 mg

Zinc 30mg

Pycnogenol 25 mg

Co–enzyme Q 10 400mg

Astragalus 50 mg

Lycopene 20mg

The DO NOT List

As with any DO list, I need to also provide you with a DO NOT list. These are foods, activities, psychological states, and substances that you should be avoiding as much as possible if you are interested in trying to prevent cancer, and many other nasty diseases.

This is a very short list, and I am sure after reading this book, you will have learned to have a personalized more complete list, but here is a short DO NOT list for cancer in particular:

Tobacco (first and second hand) smoke and chewing tobacco

Sugar particularly processed sugar

Meat, chicken, fish

Some artificial sweeteners

Excessive quantities of caffeine (coffee, tea, coke)

Various artificial colorings

Full fat Dairy products

All fried oils (and bad fats such as saturated, hydrogenated oils,

trans-fatty acids found in animal
products)

Alcohol in excess

Pesticides

Chemical dyes used in cosmetics, hair
dyes, etc

Obesity

Yo-yo dieting

Stress

Less than 30 minutes a day
exercise

Unresolved repressed emotions

Sleep deprivation

Reducing Stress When Fighting Cancer

It is well known that stress and distress contribute to the detriment of the immune system. When you have cancer, the last thing you want to do is put any extra burden on the immune system.

First of all, this is the system that is hopefully going to rally the body's defenses and get you to overcome the disease.

Secondly, if you are having traditional chemotherapy, its major effect is on the immune system, usually to render it ineffective for a while until the chemicals have killed the bad cells we call cancer. The hope is that afterwards, it will come back and do its normal job of defending the body from other invaders.

Distress is bad stress, the kind that does you no good. It does not prepare you for flight or fight. It just drains your system of energy and the effectiveness of the immune system.

In cancer therapy and prevention, it is important to eliminate distress from the body's repertoire. In other sections of this book, we discuss this at length. We discuss the use of meditation, relaxation response, aromatherapy, herbs, and the like in eliminating this kind of stressor.

Eliminating stress can be as easy as the aromatherapy treatment where you smell the roses; a trip to the seashore where you take in the sea air; or the mountains and the fresh smell of pine.

In any event, working at eliminating bad stress called distress from your life will go a long way to preventing cancer, and a whole host of other problems.

CHAPTER 7

HEART HEALTH

Exercise is of course a primary aspect of keeping a healthy heart. There are also many things in our diets that can lead to cardiovascular health.

I would briefly like to mention some heart healthy foods, and then introduce some of the traditional ways of testing to see if you're heart is healthy.

In this book, we will reveal many kinds of foods and diets that are heart healthy.

Heart Disease

It is well known that heart disease is the number one killer of Americans. There are several things that can be done to prevent heart disease or to modify it once it has been established. High blood pressure and high serum lipids (cholesterol) can cause various aspects of heart disease and or make various other parts of heart disease worse.

There are a number of medications which are utilized to control blood pressure, high lipid levels, arrhythmias and other aspects of heart disease. There are also many dietary and lifestyle changes that can be done that will help modify heart disease, or prevent it from occurring.

Diet and Heart Disease

There is a significant relationship between diet and heart disease that is statistically seen in various countries. Cultures that consume less meat, more fish, and more fruits and more vegetables have significantly lower deaths from heart disease.

There is also strong correlation between diets that are high in fats and a high rate of death from heart disease. Countries like Japan that have a much higher intake of anti oxidants and bioflavonoids have the lowest rates from heart disease.

Of course, we all know that cigarette smoking is a major factor in causing heart disease. Consequently we North Americans could save over a hundred billion dollars a year if we ate better, got more exercise, had less stress and stopped smoking.

Heart Protective Foods

America's love affair with fast food has extended too many aspects of the American diet. Unfortunately, this health-less diet has most of the nutrients removed, which are replaced with harmful preservatives and additives, putting people at risk of serious health conditions, particularly heart disease.

This particularly happens when food is refined and processed for canning, long shelf life, and even for many frozen foods. Besides having less nutrition, and costing more, refined foods tend to have less fiber, more fat, and more sweets.

As many studies have shown cultures that eat large amounts of fresh fruits and vegetables in their whole state, have a lower cancer risk as well as less heart disease.

It is believed that this is because whole foods tend to have all the necessary enzymes, minerals, vitamins, amino acids, and other nutritional substances that are needed to combat various diseases.

Beans – these are packed with heart healthy nutrients including antioxidants, magnesium, folate, and fiber.

Edamame (green soybeans) – can be a tasty healthy snack. They're high in protein and can lower triglyceride levels. They also contain plenty of fiber, which also lowers your cholesterol. Most beans are good for you especially soybeans.

Resveratrol/Grape Seed Extract/Red Wine –these are antioxidants and may protect the artery walls. They also can boost the HDL (or good cholesterol). If you drink alcohol, a few tablespoons of red wine a day may be a heart healthy choice. If you don't drink alcohol, resveratrol and various catechins, can be taken in pill form.

Omegas – Omega-3, 6, and 9 – are known to be heart healthy foods, as are EPA and DHA. Omega-3 lowers the risk of rhythm disorders like atrial fibrillation, tachycardia, etc. They are also known to lower the blood triglycerides and reduce inflammation. These good fats are available in capsule form, bottles of oil and from tuna and salmon.

Extra virgin olive oil – can be used to replace foods like butter and other saturated fats. Extra virgin olive oil will help lower your cholesterol. The Polyphenols contained in the first press of olives is especially rich in heart healthy antioxidants. Cold pressed oils are healthier than other commercial methods of pressing oils.

Nuts – these high protein foods are especially helpful in providing the body omega-3's, fiber and monounsaturated fats. For example, walnuts can lower cholesterol and reduce inflammation in the arteries of the heart. Walnuts are also high in protein, vitamin E, fiber, monounsaturated fats, protein, and plant sterols. Almonds can help lower the LDL (bad) cholesterol and are a tasty way of doing it.

Soy protein – comes in many different forms, and it is an important meat/protein alternative. Tofu is found in many different forms, and can be formulated to taste like most anything you want. In most Asian grocery stores, you can find a multitude of varieties that will satisfy any taste bud. These are full of minerals, fiber, and polyunsaturated fats.

Yams – sweet potatoes – these are healthy substitute for regular potatoes as they have a low glycemic index. They will not spike your blood sugar like regular potatoes. Regular baked potatoes are also considered a good food, but not as heart healthy as sweet potatoes. Yams also have Vitamin A, lycopene, and plenty of fiber.

Oranges/lemons/limes–these citrus fruits – contain the antioxidant hesperidin. This is believed to improve blood vessel function. Oranges also contain potassium, which is necessary for proper heart function, if it is depleted by a diuretic medication, which is often used for high blood pressure.

Carrots – these contain lots of soluble fiber, which is necessary to fight cholesterol. They also will help control blood sugar levels even though they contain a lot of natural sugar.

Swiss Chard – is a vegetable, which is rich in minerals, potassium, and magnesium all healthy for your heart. Besides the fiber that this dark green leafy vegetable has, it also contains Vitamin A and two antioxidants: Lutein and zeaxanthin, which are known to help the heart.

Whole Grains – are heart healthy. For example, oatmeal can help the heart by lowering LDL (bad cholesterol) and help keep your blood sugar levels stable by filling you up. Oat bran is an excellent source of fiber, which also helps the heart.

Do not use the pre-boiled, instant oats, as these highly processed foods do not have all of these good benefits. Barley and Spelt are other whole grains that with their fiber can also help lower cholesterol levels especially when cooked whole and added to soups, burgers, etc

Plant Sterols – these are the healthy part of many vegetables. The sterols and stanols are extracted from the plants and work by blocking cholesterol absorption in the digestive tract, and thereby lowering the LDL levels.

Flax – this is often been called a miracle food because of its ingredients, which are extremely good for the heart. This seed has fiber, phytochemicals (lignans), and ALA (another omega-3 fatty acid). ALA is converted to EPA and DHA, which are the more powerful omega-3.

Probiotics – they're many forms of these friendly bacteria that can help the heart by keeping your gastrointestinal tract in order. In addition, if you get your friendly bacteria from low fat yogurt, it has plenty of calcium, potassium and other nutrients that are healthy to the heart.

Fruits – many fruits have antioxidants that help protect blood vessels. For example, cherries have anthocyanins–a powerful antioxidant. Pomegranates also contain a number of powerful antioxidants. Blueberries have anthocyanins; ellagic acid, lutein, Vitamin C, beta-carotene, magnesium, potassium, fiber, and folate (Vitamin B) and are all heart healthy.

Chili Peppers – although one has to accustom oneself to it, using chili powder on food has been shown to lower insulin levels in obese individuals. This will help your heart; however, if you have a sensitive stomach you should be cautious.

Fiber – the plant substance that is not digested is very important for the well-being of your heart. It is recommended that you have at least thirty grams of fiber a day. Although we do not know all the benefits of fiber, we do know that it acts like a giant broom that sweeps the intestines clean.

This prevents the absorption of some fat and many toxins that would otherwise be absorbed into the body from the intestinal tract. The decrease in total fats will protect your heart. Besides fresh fruit and vegetables, whole grains such as barley, oats, millet, wheat, corn, quinoa, rice and amaranth also have heart protective qualities.

Whole grains and legumes provide most of the fiber that is needed for a healthy heart and also provide a rich source of protein and complex carbohydrates. As you will see throughout this book whole grains and legumes form an important basis for a healthy diet.

If one insists on eating a processed diet, one can add the necessary fiber to the diet by taking tablespoons of raw wheat bran, oat bran, psyllium seed or psyllium husk. Remember not to add significant amounts of bran or psyllium too rapidly to your diet. When you are not used to a lot of fiber it can cause bloating, gas, and loose stool, so go slow.

As we already mentioned, countries that have high intakes of fresh fruits and vegetables have a lower rate of heart disease. Some researchers correlate this with the increased amounts of Vitamin E and antioxidants that are present in fresh fruits and vegetables. These antioxidants are a primary defense against damage that otherwise occurs to the blood vessels particularly of the heart by free radicals.

Polyphenols, Folic acid, various minerals, Chlorophyll, Thiocyanates, Dithiolethiones and Sulforaphane are found in fresh fruits and vegetables. These have protective qualities, and produce enzymes, (i.e. glutathione) which also have protective value to the heart and blood vessels.

Soybeans and Lecithin

Soybeans are a very good source of protein, are relatively low in fat and they contain many nutrients, which are helpful to the heart. A 1/2-cup serving of boiled soybeans contains 150 calories, 9g of unsaturated fat, 1 g saturated fat, 5g of fiber, and 14g of protein.

Soybeans contain iron, magnesium, lecithin, choline, and other vitamins and minerals, as well as phytoestrogens. These occupy the estrogen receptor sites causing a decrease in the amount of LVL cholesterol in the person taking soybeans in the diet.

Various other chemicals found in soybeans are also indicated in lowering serum cholesterol. Thytic acid binds to iron and increases copper absorption in the human body. Adequate copper leads to a normal cholesterol level. Soy also increases the production of bile salts, which uses up cholesterol in the serum, and therefore, can be excreted in the feces.

There are a variety of soy products, which will be presented in this book. Soy is a very universal product because the protein in it can be chopped, cooked, spun, and various other procedures so that it can be made into many different products. High and low fat tofu, soymilk tempeh, and miso are only a few of the many soy products that can be used in a heart healthy diet.

Salt

Although there is currently much debate about the use of salt in a heart healthy diet now in the late 1990's, there are a few facts about sodium, which need to be mentioned in any discussion on healthy hearts.

We do need some sodium in our diet. It helps to regulate muscle contractions, nerve stimulation, appropriate fluid balance in the cells, digestion of food in the stomach, and the absorption of calcium and other minerals into the blood.

Eating the appropriate fresh vegetables and fruits will provide sufficient sodium to maintain these functions. Eating a typically American highly processed diet will push you well above the 500 to 2500 milligrams per day total daily need for sodium.

The average American consumes about fifteen pounds of salt every year or about sixty five times what is needed by the body. This, of course, leads to high blood pressure, fluid retention, and migraines among other problems.

Besides processed food, you will also find salt in beer, baking soda and baking powder, cough syrups, anti acids, laxatives, prepared meats, sodas, various preservatives, and pickles.

Although current research shows that you likely do not need to eliminate all added salt from the diet you definitely do not need to eat heavily salted foods. There are many other spices and herbs which can flavor food. If you are eating whole fresh foods that need salt, then ensure it is minimal.

Garlic

Garlic can help the diet in three ways:

☑ It can lower serum lipids (fats)
☑ It can moderate blood clotting
☑ It can control blood pressure

Studies show that people who consume large amounts of garlic have lower cholesterol levels and particularly lower LDL levels. Routine use of garlic will continually decrease the LDL levels and increase the HDL levels, which is protective against heart disease.

Garlic appears to slow down internal cholesterol production, and decrease the negative effects of increased dietary cholesterol intake. It has also been shown that garlic moves the stored fat levels from the tissues thereby helping to get excess cholesterol eliminated.

Garlic and Blood Pressure

In Asia, garlic has been used for the treatment of high blood pressure for centuries. It appears that garlic carries out its action of lowering blood pressure by relaxing smooth muscles, or regulating the production of a particular hormone.

Garlic and Clotting

It appears that garlic compounds help blood clots dissolve faster and improve the fluidity of blood. Garlic moderates the blood clotting time, and other aspects of the clotting cascade. Eating garlic will help prevent the blood clotting that can lead to coronary thrombosis and result in a myocardial infarction (heart attack).

Studies have also shown that garlic can reduce the degree of blockage in the arteries. There has also been a reversal of atherosclerosis measured with the intake of garlic. When eaten raw, the use of cooked cloves, or by taking one of the many extracts in pill or capsule form, one can enjoy the heart health benefits of garlic. Use caution in social situations as garlic does have a pungent odor if used in excess. I recall one patient who took my advice to the extreme and consumed 5 bulbs of garlic per day. When I entered the exam room, it was all I could do to not faint from the overwhelming odor.

Alcohol

Too much alcohol is bad for the heart. Chronic alcohol intake depletes the body of magnesium, which can lead to heart disease. Studies have also shown that increased alcohol intake can lead to higher blood pressure readings. Alcohol is known to show increased risk of death from cancer and cirrhosis of the liver.

That said, recent medical research has shown that a little bit of red wine is beneficial to the heart. It appears that the positive benefits of wine, particularly red wine, are in the reduction of the activity of clotting agents in the blood. There are other natural agents that will do similar things.

The epidemiological studies indicate that the health benefits in groups studied, such as the French, did not rest with the wine alone. The lower rates of heart disease were accompanied by higher intakes of fruits and vegetables.

It seems a little bit (two tablespoons) of red wine several times a week, in addition to large amounts of fruits, vegetables, and grains may be beneficial to your heart health.

Water

Water is essential for a heart healthy diet. One should drink eight to ten large glasses of water daily. It has no calories, no caffeine, no sugar, no fat and no preservatives. It is needed for the biochemistry of the body to function properly, and to flush out toxins that your body has acquired.

One needs to drink sufficient water so that dehydration does not adversely affect the heart. Dehydration can cause abnormal heartbeats, electrolyte imbalances, kidney and bladder problems, and it can be a contributing factor to a number of common diseases.

Water is essential for good digestion and elimination of toxins through sweat, urine, and feces. It helps rid the blood of excess fat, and consequently helps the heart stay healthy. It is important to drink water that is clean and without contamination by heavy metals, benzene and other carcinogenic toxins. Caution with some of the sales pitches for water filters, as some of these can eliminate all the minerals that water has.

Heart Testing:

Electrocardiograms

There are electrical pulses given out by your heart that can be recorded on a piece of paper. This is commonly known as an electrocardiogram or an ECG/EKG.

This tells us if there are irregular rhythms (arrhythmias), evidence of strain in the heart (heart attacks and or almost heart attacks) and various other more subtle abnormalities in the heartbeat.

Stress tests

Stress tests are a method of telling whether you're heart can tolerate exercise. In this test, you are put on a treadmill with all the appropriate connections to your heart, like a cardiogram. As you exercise on the treadmill it records your heart rate and electrical impulses.

This allows the physician to determine if, while you exercise, there are any abnormalities. You will probably hear your physician talk about a Bruce protocol. This is a generally accepted method of speeding up the treadmill to make you exercise along statistically accepted parameters.

Stress tests can also be performed without having to make you run on a treadmill. This is often done for people who have already known cardiovascular disease, people who are grossly overweight, people who have arthritic changes and cannot run on a treadmill, and the elderly who might have a heart attack if they ran on a treadmill.

These tests are done with persantine and various other combinations of scanning materials: Persantine stress test, persantine thallium stress test, persantine cardiolite stress test, and persantine nuclear stress test, etc. For these tests, you lie down and enjoy the peace and quiet during the test.

Cardiac CT

This is a CT (computerized tomography) test of your heart. Many pictures are taken and then correlated to determine if there are calcium deposits and/or other signs that you may have heart disease.

Lab Testing

Inflammation plays a central role in the process of atherosclerosis, in which fatty deposits clog, narrow, and restrict blood flow. Measuring CRP, one of the popularized lab tests, alone won't tell your doctor your risk of heart disease but is a good start.

The following are a list of cardiovascular tests to recommend having done at your doctor's office or lab. Some are easy to get, others are expensive and many labs do not provide.

- ☑ C-reactive protein
- ☑ Fibrinogen
- ☑ Homocysteine
- ☑ Cholesterol test
- ☑ Lipoprotein (a)
- ☑ Natriuretic peptides

C Reactive Protein (CRP) Testing

This test is an inflammation marker! It tests to see if one has inflammation in the body. It is NOT specific, much like the ESR (erythrocite sedimentation rate).

Fibrinogen Test

Fibrinogen is a protein in your blood that helps blood clot. However, too much fibrinogen can cause a clot to form in an artery, leading to a heart attack or stroke.

Having too much fibrinogen may also mean that you have atherosclerosis. It may also worsen existing injury to artery walls.

Your doctor may check your fibrinogen level if you have an increased risk of heart disease. Smoking, inactivity, drinking too much alcohol, and taking supplemental estrogen — whether from birth control pills or hormone therapy, may increase your fibrinogen level.

A normal fibrinogen level is considered to be between 200 and 400 mg/L depending on the labs, it's better to be near 200.

Homocysteine Test

Homocysteine is a substance your body uses to make protein and to build and maintain tissue. But too much homocysteine may increase your risk of stroke, certain types of heart disease, and disease of the blood vessels of the arms, legs and feet (peripheral artery disease).

Cholesterol Tests

A cholesterol test, also called a lipid panel or lipid profile, measures the fats (lipids) in your blood. The measurements can indicate your risk of having a heart attack or other heart disease. The test typically includes measurements of:

☑ Total cholesterol –This is a sum of your blood's cholesterol content. A high level can put you at increased risk of heart disease.

☑ Low-density lipoprotein (LDL) cholesterol – This is sometimes called the "bad" cholesterol. Too much of it in your blood causes the accumulation of fatty deposits (plaques) in your arteries (atherosclerosis), which reduces blood flow. These plaques sometimes rupture and lead to major heart and vascular problems.

☑ High-density lipoprotein (HDL) cholesterol – This is sometimes called the "good" cholesterol because it helps carry away LDL cholesterol, keeping arteries open and your blood flowing more freely.

☑ Triglycerides – High triglyceride levels usually mean you regularly eat more calories than you burn. High levels increase your risk of heart disease.

Natriuretic Peptides

Atrial natriuretic peptide (ANP) is a powerful vasodilator, and a protein polypeptide hormone secreted by heart muscle cells. It is involved in the homeostatic control of the body's water, potassium, fat and sodium. These natriuretic peptides are released by muscle cells in the upper chambers of the heart, in response to high blood pressure. ANP reduces the water, sodium, and adipose loads on the circulatory system, which in turn reduces blood pressure

Used in conjunction with other clinical information, measurement of B-type natriuretic peptide (BNP) can help determine whether a patient's shortness of breath (dyspnea) is caused by congestive heart failure. This laboratory test has become a valuable and quick method for diagnostic work-up of patients presenting to the emergency department with acute dyspnea.

We are going to explore the necessary testing, and the new advancements for treatment and my protocol. The possible causes of CVD (cardiovascular disease) are numerous, including epigenetic, genetics, dietary, lifestyle, lack of exercise, and just your belief systems and identities.

CHAPTER 8

METABOLIC SYNDROME

Metabolic syndrome is the name for a group of risk factors that raise your risk for heart disease and other health problems, such as diabetes and stroke.

The term "metabolic" refers to the biochemical processes involved in the body's normal functioning. Risk factors are traits, conditions, or habits that increase your chance of developing a disease.

Metabolic Risk Factors

The five conditions described below are metabolic risk factors. You may have any one of these risk factors alone; however, they tend to occur together. You must have at least three metabolic risk factors to win the prize and receive a diagnosis of metabolic syndrome.

- ☑ **A Large Waistline** –This also is called having an apple shape, or abdominal obesity. Those with excess abdominal fat are at a much greater risk for heart disease than those with excess fat in other areas of the body, such as on the hips.

- ☑ **A High Triglyceride Level** – is a type of fat found in the blood, and it can lead to a heart attack.

- ☑ **A Low HDL Cholesterol Level** – HDL is called the good" cholesterol, because it helps remove cholesterol from your arteries. A low HDL cholesterol level raises your risk for heart disease.

- ☑ **High Blood Pressure** – The systolic (top one) BP is a reading of the force of blood pushing against the walls of your arteries as your heart pumps blood. The diastolic (lower reading) BP indicates the pressure on the blood vessels when the heart is to be resting.

- ☑ If it is too high, it means that your heart is not resting (from the pressure) when it is supposed to. If your blood pressure rises and stays high over time, it can damage your heart, blood vessels, and lead to plaque buildup.

☑ **High Fasting Blood Sugar** - high blood sugar can be an early sign of diabetes. A fasting blood sugar and a Hemoglobin A1c best test this. These two tests tell us what the status of the blood sugar is and has been for the last 30-60 days.

Overview of Metabolic Syndrome

Your risk for heart disease, diabetes, and stroke increases with the number of metabolic risk factors you have. Generally, a person with a metabolic syndrome is twice as likely to develop heart disease, and five times as likely to develop diabetes as someone who doesn't have metabolic syndrome.

There are other risk factors besides those described that will increase your risk for heart disease. For example, if you have a high LDL cholesterol level (bad cholesterol) this will signal the collection of fats in your arteries and subsequently heart disease. If you smoke, you are at high risk for developing heart disease.

The chance of developing metabolic syndrome is closely linked to being overweight combined with a lack of physical activity. If you are insulin resistant, you could have an increased risk for metabolic syndrome.

Insulin resistance is a condition in which the body is not able to properly use insulin, a hormone that helps move blood sugar into cells where it is used to produce energy.

Outlook

As a result of a rise in obesity, metabolic syndrome is becoming more common. It is predicted that in the future, metabolic syndrome will overtake smoking alone as the leading risk factor for heart disease.

Lifestyle changes can prevent or delay the development of metabolic syndrome. A healthy lifestyle is a lifelong commitment. Successfully controlling metabolic syndrome requires long-term effort on your part while working with your doctor and other health care providers.

CHAPTER 9

FERTILITY

Male Fertility Health

With male fertility concerns rising over the years, there have also been a number of discussions on natural supplements that can be taken to boost the fertility of men. Various changes in lifestyle, stress, pollution, technology etc. have all in some way or other contributed to lowering fertility in men.

Causes of Male Infertility:

Male infertility can be caused due to various reasons, such as:

- ☑ Stress

- ☑ Sperm disorders

- ☑ Retrograde ejaculation

- ☑ Genetic problems

- ☑ Obstruction in the passage where the sperm must pass

- ☑ Medical conditions that may cause impotency

- ☑ Hormonal problems

- ☑ Alcohol Consumption

- ☑ Smoking

- ☑ Exposure to excessive heat

These are the most commonly seen causes, although there are others. While some of the reasons listed above need medical intervention there are some causes that can be tackled with the help of natural sources too. There are claims that pumpkin seeds (and oil) may boost the overall health of the reproductive system and improve sperm count naturally.

Pumpkin Seeds

Pumpkin seeds are high in zinc and have some vital fatty acids that work well in boosting the male reproductive system and thereby increase fertility. For men suffering from a low sperm count the hunt for help stops at pumpkin seeds.

Zinc is vital for the production of testosterone and for a healthy prostate gland to produce healthy and potent sperm and semen (the fluid the sperm travels in). Thus by introducing pumpkin seeds in your diet you can improve your sperm count, have healthier sperm, and maintain the right level of testosterone. The dosage should always be discussed with your doctor as zinc intake can cause toxicity in the body.

Pumpkin seeds are often called one of "nature's perfect foods" as they have the right nutritional content balance. Vitamins carbohydrates, amino acids, calcium, phosphorous, zinc, potassium, and fatty acids are present in them.

The fatty acids present in pumpkin seeds go a long way in improving the fluidity and mobility of sperm in the semen. It helps by thinning the sperm membrane that, in turn, betters the chance of fertilizing the female egg. You can have about _ cup of pumpkin seeds per day to boost the overall health of the male reproductive system.

Lifestyle Changes

1. Apart from pumpkin seeds there are some lifestyle changes, you need to incorporate for a holistic treatment of your fertility issues.

2. Secondly, drastically cut down on your alcohol intake.

3. Smoking is a big no-no for men suffering from reduced fertility.

4. Eat a healthy diet with the right nutritional content.

5. Add in some form of exercise too.

Incorporate all these changes in your lifestyle, and you would no longer suffer from fertility problems.

Female Fertility Health

Frustration can occur when a couple has sex like clockwork during ovulation and yet pregnancy does not occur. Taking charge of your fertility goes much farther than just having sexual intercourse.

Causes of Female Infertility

Female infertility can be caused due to various reasons like

- ☑ Age – a woman's fertility begins to decline after age 35
- ☑ Problems with ovulation – affects 33% to 50% of all women
- ☑ Problems with the hypothalamus or pituitary gland
- ☑ Blocked fallopian tubes
- ☑ Cervical mucus problems
- ☑ Endometriosis
- ☑ Polycystic Ovarian Syndrome
- ☑ Cancer Treatments

Lifestyle Changes to increase fertility

1. **Shape Up** – Staying healthy is important to your general well–being, and it becomes much more important when you are trying to conceive. Poor health is one of the major causes of infertility. There are a number of other causes of infertility, which we will look at shortly.

2. **Avoid Processed Food** – If you eat a lot of processed food or takeout food you should eliminate, or at the very least cut back. They offer little to no nutritional value, which you need more than ever if you are trying to become pregnant.

3. **Exercise at Least Three Times Per Week** – Kick start your fertility with a good exercise program. You should exercise at minimum of three times a week for at least 30 minutes. Cardiovascular exercise helps the blood circulate, which leads to better blood flow in the reproductive organs.

4. **Stop Smoking and Avoid Alcohol** – If your smoke, you need to stop, because it can affect your fertility. If you have the occasional drink it won't matter, but if you have more than three drinks a day, or you binge drink, you need to quit, because it can lead to infertility.

CHAPTER 10

FLU SHOTS

According to the CDC the "flu shot" is generally an inactivate vaccine, containing killed virus that is given with a needle, usually in the arm. The flu shot is approved for use in people older than 6 months, including healthy people and those individuals with chronic medical conditions.

There are three different flu shots available:

☑ A regular flu shot approved for people ages 6 months and older.
☑ A high-dose flu shot approved for people 65 and older.
☑ An intradermal flu shot approved for people 18 to 64 years of age.

The nasal-spray flu vaccine, a vaccine made with live, weakened flu viruses that are given as a nasal spray, is sometimes called LAIV for "Live Attenuated Influenza Vaccine". The viruses in the nasal spray vaccine do not cause the flu. LAIV is approved for use in healthy people between the ages of 2 through 49 years of age who are not pregnant.

Seasonal flu vaccines protect against the three influenza viruses that research indicates will be most common during the upcoming season.

The viruses in the vaccine can change each year based on international surveillance and scientists' estimations about which types and strains of viruses will circulate in a given year.

About 2 weeks after vaccination, antibodies that provide protection against the influenza viruses in the vaccine, develop in the body.

When to Get Vaccinated

The CDC recommends that people get their seasonal flu vaccine as soon as the vaccine becomes available in their community. Vaccination before December is best since this timing ensures that protective antibodies are in place before flu activity is typically at its highest.

The CDC encourages people to get vaccinated throughout the flu season, which can begin as early as October and last as late as May. Over the course of the flu season, many different influenza viruses can circulate at different times and in different places.

As long as flu viruses are still spreading in the community, vaccination can provide protective benefit.

Where to Get Vaccinated

Flu vaccine shipments begin in August, and continue throughout September and October until all the vaccine is distributed. Doctors and nurses are encouraged to begin vaccinating their patients as soon as flu vaccine is available in their area, even as early as August. See your doctor or nurse for your flu vaccine or seek out other locations where vaccine is being offered.

Who Should Get Vaccinated

On February 24, 2010, vaccine experts voted that everyone 6 months and older should get a flu vaccine each year starting with the 2010–2011 influenza season. CDC's Advisory Committee on Immunization Practices (ACIP) voted for "universal" flu vaccinations within the U.S. to expand protection against the flu to more people.

While everyone should get a flu vaccine each flu season, it's especially important that the following groups get vaccinated either because they are at high risk of having serious flu-related complications or because they live with or care for people at high risk for developing flu-related complications:

Pregnant women

1. Children younger than 5, but especially children younger than 2 years old

2. People 50 years of age and older

3. People of any age with certain chronic medical conditions.
4. People who live in nursing homes and other long-term care facilities People who live with or care for those at high risk for complications from flu, including:

    • Health care workers.

- Household contacts of persons at high risk for complications from the flu.

- Household contacts and out of home caregivers of children less than 6 months of age (these children are too young to be vaccinated).

Who Should Not Be Vaccinated

There are some people who should not get a flu vaccine without first consulting a physician. These include:

- People who have a *severe* allergy to chicken eggs.

- People who have had a severe reaction to an influenza vaccination.

- People who developed Guillain Barre Syndrome (GBS) within 6 weeks of getting an influenza vaccine.

- Children younger than 6 months of age (influenza vaccine is not approved for this age group).

- People who have a moderate-to-severe illness with a fever who should wait until they recover to get vaccinated.

Vaccine Effectiveness

The ability of a flu vaccine to protect a person depends on the age and health status of the person getting the vaccine, and the similarity or "match" between the viruses or virus in the vaccine and those in circulation.

Vaccine Side Effects – What to Expect

Different side effects can be associated with the flu shot and LAIV.
The viruses in the flu shot are killed, so <u>you cannot get the flu from a flu shot</u>. Some minor side effects that could occur are:

- Soreness, redness, or swelling where the shot was given

- Fever (low grade)

- Aches

If these problems occur, they begin soon after the shot and usually last 1 to 2 days. Almost all people who receive influenza vaccine have no serious problems from it.

The nasal spray vaccine is called LAIV or FluMist®. The viruses in the nasal-spray vaccine are weakened and do not cause severe symptoms often associated with influenza illness.

In children, side effects from LAIV (FluMist®) can include:

- Runny nose

- Wheezing

- Headache

- Vomiting

- Muscle ache

- Fever

In adults, side effects from LAIV (FluMist®) can include:
- Runny nose

- Headache

- Sore throat

- Cough

Influenza Facts

The symptoms of influenza appear suddenly and often include:

✓ Fever of 100 °F (37.8 °C) to 104 °F (40 °C), which can reach 106 °F (41.1 °C) when symptoms first develop. Fever is usually continuous, but it may come and go.

✓ Shaking chills.

✓ Body aches and severe muscle pain, commonly in the back, arms, or legs.

✓ Headache & Pain when you move your eyes.

✓ A general feeling of sickness (malaise) and loss of appetite.

✓ A dry cough, runny nose, and dry or sore throat. You may not notice these during the first few days of the illness when other symptoms are more severe. As fever goes away, these symptoms usually become more evident.

Tips for Preventing the Flu

There are no known cures for colds and flu; therefore, prevention must be your goal. Keeping your body as healthy as you can is the best way of preventing the flu. Remember, antibiotics have NO EFFECT on the flu. Other pills only somewhat dull the symptoms.

#1 Wash Your Hands

Most cold and flu viruses are spread by direct contact. Someone who has the flu sneezes onto their hand, and then touches the telephone, the computer keyboard, a kitchen glass, keypads on debit machines, etc. The germs can live for hours -- in some cases weeks, only to be picked up by the next person who touches the same object. So wash your hands often, and use hand sanitizer.

#2 Don't Touch Your Face

Cold and flu viruses enter your body through the eyes, nose, or mouth. Touching their faces is the major way children catch colds, and the main way children pass colds on to their parents.

#3 Drink Plenty of Fluids

Water flushes your system, washing out the poisons as it rehydrates you. A typical, healthy adult needs eight 8-ounce glasses of fluids each day (three liters).

How can you tell if you're getting enough liquid? If the color of your urine runs close to clear, you're getting enough. If it's deep yellow, you need more fluids. When A/C is used, it's a good idea to increase the fluids even more.

#4 Get Fresh Air

A regular dose of fresh air is important, especially in cold weather when central heating dries you out and makes your body more vulnerable to cold and flu viruses. Also, during cold weather more people stay indoors, which means more germs are circulating in crowded, dry rooms.

#5 Take Vitamin C

Taking 500mg of vitamin C twice a day will help ward off viral infections. There are many other antioxidants like Vitamin C that can help, but Vitamin C is cheap and well tolerated by most. Orange juice is a good source. L-Lysine (an amino acid) in doses of 1000mg+ per day has a similar effect. A Canadian product that is an extract of ginseng (Cold-FX) has been shown in clinical trials to prevent and/or stop colds and flu, if taken in recommended doses.

#6 Do Aerobic Exercise Regularly

Aerobic exercise speeds up the heart to pump larger quantities of blood; makes you breathe faster to help transfer oxygen from your lungs to your blood, and makes you sweat once your body heats up. These exercises help increase the body's natural virus-killing cells.

#7 Eat Foods Containing Phytochemicals

"Phyto" means plants, and the natural chemicals in plants give the vitamins in food a supercharged boost. Eat dark green, red, and yellow vegetables and fruits.

#8 Eat Yogurt

Some studies have shown that eating a few tablespoons a day of low-fat yogurt can reduce your susceptibility to colds by 25%. Researchers believe the beneficial bacteria in yogurt may stimulate production of immune system substances that fight disease.

#9 Don't Smoke

Statistics show that smokers get more severe colds, more frequent ones, and influenza. Even being around smoke profoundly zaps the immune system. Smoke dries out your nasal passages and paralyzes cilia.

These are the delicate hairs that line the mucous membranes in your nose and lungs, and with their wavy movements, sweep cold and flu viruses out of the nasal passages.

Experts contend that one cigarette can paralyze cilia for as long as 30 to 40 minutes. One hour in a smoky environment, even if you don't smoke, can rob you of millions of white blood cells that could have helped you fight off the flu.

#10 Relax

If you can teach yourself to relax, you can activate your immune system on demand. There's evidence that when you put your relaxation skills into action, your interleukins -- leaders in the immune system response against cold and flu viruses -- increase in the bloodstream.

Train yourself to picture an image you find pleasant or calming. Do this 20 minutes a day for several months. Keep in mind, relaxation is a learnable skill, but it is not doing nothing, or watching TV, or listening to music. You don't have to join a cult to learn relaxation techniques.

Hindu, Buddhist, Christian & Muslim religions all have their meditative techniques. Herbert Benson MD proved that by merely closing the eyes and thinking the number 'one' over and over for 20 minutes twice a day, that immune system improvements and decreased blood pressure could be seen.

#11 Cut Alcohol Consumption

Heavy alcohol use destroys the liver, the body's primary filtering system, which means that germs of all kinds won't leave your body as fast. The result is heavier drinkers are more prone to initial infections as well as secondary complications.

Alcohol also dehydrates the body -- it takes more fluids from your system than it puts in. A couple of tablespoons of red wine a day may help your heart and your immune system—any more and the health benefits are lost.

#12 Get Sleep

Try to get sleep every night. Ideally you should get 8 hours of sleep, but at least take naps when you can instead of watching TV, DVD's etc. Sleep boosts your immune system too.

CHAPTER 11

FAITH HEALING

Once, while still in medical school, I traveled with one of my fellow med students to do some medical volunteer work in Asia. En-route we visited one of his friends who practiced medicine in Bagio, Philippines.

For me, this was an interesting side trip, as I had never been there and enjoyed seeing his friends' hospital. We helped him out with some of his patients, which left him with more free time to spend with us. The patients respected his abilities and we two Canadian med students intrigued them.

Our doctor friend was trained in Internal Medicine in Canada, and he carried on a traditional practice of that specialty. We saw lots of people with diabetes, rheumatoid arthritis, hypertension and cancer. What intrigued both of us were the patients who mentioned that they also would regularly see one of the local faith healers to "ensure that they got better". When we first asked our friend about this, he shrugged it off. When we insisted in knowing what this was all about, he explained their local phenomenon.

Apparently, in this lovely mountainous vacation resort area of the Philippines, a number of faith healers developed their base operations. Some were known for their miraculous healing, while others were well known for taking the money of the sick and making people believe that they had been treated.

Our friend told us the basis for most was to ensure that the 'patient' had a strong faith in religion. When the patient had faith, the faith healer could tap into it, and heal their disease. With their techniques, psychic surgery was often performed. This entailed removing tumors, ulcers, and evil spirits that otherwise needed strong antipsychotic medications.

These "surgeries" were very popular and left no scar. Obviously, this intrigued us, two young med students, and we bugged our friend to take us to see these healers. He resisted a lot, but finally gave in and arranged for us to see several including a chap called Jun Labo.

The Role of Faith in Healing

This is the extreme in faith and healing. One also sees this type of faith healing in many of the traditions practiced by the Native American Tribes. The Shaman or other healer is called to invoke the spirits of ancestors and others, to rid the patient of their illness and to regain their health.

What one finds in ALL aspects of medicine is some form of faith coming into the healing process. In Western Medicine we call upon our academic gods, to physiologically rid our patients of the disease that have inhabited them.

We tend to shun any reference to prayer or religion having much to do with the healing process unless you are associated with a religiously affiliated hospital or other institution. Until recently, or at least in the last 50 years, there were virtual 'hangings' of western physicians who would even mention the strength of prayer in healing their patients.

That rather strict division of medicine and faith has softened. Now it is accepted that one can influence the recovery of themselves when there is a belief in a higher power through prayer, or by your loved ones praying for you. Having strong psychological support systems is scientifically proven to aid in the recovery of patients. Included in these support systems are religion, prayer, and faith.

Some people have even shown that prayer can speed up recovery, and reverse certain conditions that were otherwise thought to be hopeless. Some have shown just the opposite. The truth is still up for grabs as to the actual extent of what prayer and faith can physiologically do, but we do know it does something.

We also know that you can give people the same pill for the same condition and get different outcomes just by giving positive reinforcement to a patient. This is a form of faith. The patient believes that the medicine will help, and it does. The same goes for faith in ones doctor.

If a patient believes and has faith in his/her doctor the outcome of that person's treatment will be more positive, than the patient who does not have complete confidence in the competency, skill, or other abilities of their doctor.

This also applies to the doctor too. Throughout medical school we were led to believe, "have faith in what you are taught". Often this was given to us as 'gospel truth'. Over the years, this has been an effective way of imparting information to students of medicine.

Galen set forth the 'gospel truth' about the various body humors and how essential it was to treat them. We know that this and MANY other fads and theories in medicine are just bunk. We learn new things daily in medicine. It is the good doctor who keeps learning and modifying his/her practice to accommodate these changes.

Still when the doctor gives that prescription as being the right one, he must have faith that it is. Otherwise, the patient will not have the necessary faith that it will work and, as a result, it will not have the same effect.

Medicine does have an aspect of faith associated with it. However, we must sort out the beneficial aspects of faith from the hucksters who do more harm than good. When these hucksters make a person believe that the treatment is going to cure their serious disease, and that person forgoes proven treatments with other medicine, an enormous disservice occurs.

More on Faith Healers

Later in my career, I was asked by a prestigious university in the US to take a trip to Bagio, Philippines while doing some volunteer work. This is the same colorful Bagio, built on a number of hills in the 'mountainous' part of Luzon that I visited as a medical student. I was asked to visit a number of the faith healers to determine if there was any scientific basis to their claims.

Interspersed in this active Phillipino community are the dwellings of the faith healers. Some of these buildings are simple storefronts with advertisements as to their claims of faith healing out front. In many cases, the signage is bigger than the building itself.

Some are old homes that have been converted. They have comfortable waiting areas with 'treatment rooms' and 'consulting rooms' developed in the structure. There are also several facilities that look more like five star hotels with accommodations for their visitors/patients; complete with elegant waiting rooms.

I chose to spend my limited time with three different facilities. Two of the more modest converted home places, and one of the hotel-like facilities. I decided to forgo the storefront come-ons. My choice was principally based upon recommendations from locals and information I had gathered from others prior to arriving.

As a middle-aged male, I could easily pass as a potential patient. Not totally untrue, I have a family history of cardiac disease, and personally do have high blood pressure, which is well controlled with simple traditional BP medicine.

Healer #1

I presented to the first faith healers office, and was greeted by a charming young receptionist. She took my particulars and credit card, deducting a hefty sum from the latter, and ushered me into the living room of the remodeled home where comfortable seats greeted me.

After waiting 15 minutes, I was ushered into an office where the healer sat behind an impressive desk. He asked a few dutiful questions, and then informed me that after his treatment I would no longer need my blood pressure pills.

In Tagalog, which is the local language, he said a few sentences, which I was able to understand enough to hear him say 'take away disease'. He then put his hand on my forehead and pushed me back into the chair.

Then announced, I was cured. I asked if he could now take my BP, to which he responded that it would be better to wait a few hours. I did, and my BP was unchanged. I was still taking my daily pill.

Healer #2

Visit two was to a fancier old home that had been redone a bit better than the first, which had the same type of charming receptionist, who took a bigger chunk of my available credit on my credit card.

I was quickly ushered into a room, told to undress, and given a bright colored gown to put on. I was then placed in a chair resembling the one my dentist uses. The healer soon came in, and with very cold hands examined me in a manner not taught in any medical school, at least not any that I know of.

His hands whisked up and down over my body stopping every once in a while. There, he would tap my body repetitively and make a grunting noise. Then with an extremely fast motion he made a motion over my chest, and produced a wet bloody bit of tissue. He wiped my chest, and proclaimed that I was cured. I again asked my now standard question as to having him take my BP. He did and said it was normal. Later that afternoon, I confirmed that my BP was the same as it always was on medication. His treatment did not lower my BP.

Healer #3

The third place I went was one of the five star hotel facilities. I was required to stay overnight in a small, but very nicely appointed room. I was given a decent breakfast and then ushered into a conference room filled mostly with Japanese guests.

In three languages, we were told about the wonderfulness of the healer and that we would all be cured. We were told that some of us would need to stay longer than others; and that certain other treatments may be necessary, like physical therapy, and special diets. But for the most part, only treatments by the healer were necessary.

Later that afternoon, I was delivered from my room to an elegant treatment room, the envy of any physician! Lights were lowered and nice music was playing. Eventually the healer entered the room with the appearance of a magician on stage complete with flowing robes.

Even though he was not quite four feet in height, he certainly had a presence. He made noises and spoke in a language other than Tagalong. He also whisked his hands over my body like the other healer but his hands were not cold. He did a tapping motion, and when he came to my chest, he said "oh here is the problem" and promptly "removed" tissue from my chest -- a bloody, slimy bit of what appeared to be connective tissue.

He immediately proclaimed that I was cured, and no longer needed my medicine. I again asked if he would take my BP to which he looked insulted that I would doubt his word that I was cured. I checked out of my room, and away I went. Later that afternoon, I again confirmed that my BP was the same as it always was on medication. His treatment did not lower my BP.

My Healer Study

As I needed to learn more than was obvious from the treatments, I decided to return to the second healer and asked if I could pay for some more of his time for a study the university was doing. He agreed.

This faith healer, whom I will identify as Ricardo, was a 53-year-old Filipino from the local area. His father and grandfather were both faith healers. His education was through middle school in the local Catholic school. Speaking good English, Ricardo gave the impression of being a very savvy businessman and a personable individual.

I explained to him that the university was interested in learning more about faith healing and that they would like to observe him in an experiment in Singapore. After explaining the particulars, we discussed his practice.

He explained to us that there were many Asians that came to be treated who were not necessarily believers of any particular religion, but if they believed in the treatment, then they could be cured. He indicated that he was a Christian but not necessarily attached to any particular church. He said it did not matter if patients were Christians, Buddhists, Hindus, or Jews; they can all be cured.

Arrangements were made, and two months later Ricardo boarded a plane for Singapore. He was brought to one of the University Hospitals for housing and the experiment. He was provided a meal, hospital greens, and a padded cell normally used for psychiatric patients, as the only means of insuring that Ricardo had no possibility of access to any outside material or devices.

Ricardo had a nice vegetarian meal that evening and a morning breakfast. He was allowed a shower and he was observed while he dressed in his hospital greens. Arrangements were made with the local hospital for a patient with thyroid cancer to participate in the experiment.

She was similarly dressed in hospital greens. She consented to the upcoming procedure with the understanding that the usual allopathic methodology of radiation and surgery would be provided if the faith healing failed to provide any change to her status.

Ricardo entered the room and was filmed from several angles. He was wearing the short-sleeved hospital greens. He did a similar procedure as he had done to me with his hands scanning the body. He was not told what the patient had, other than the fact that she was ill. The thyroid tumor was somewhat obvious to a trained observer. At one point during the process, he 'removed' some tissue from her neck and presented it to the attending technicians.

According to observers, there was no apparent place he could have obtained material. There was no open wound or scar. The material was sent to the pathology lab, and the usual tests were performed. It showed, by DNA and tissue typing, that it was not the patients' thyroid tissue.

A scan performed later, indicated that the previous cancer was still present. No scientific explanation could be made of the tissue that he 'removed' in the experiment.

You can quickly see that some individuals may possess a gift as a faith healer that patients can benefit from. However, without scientific proof it will remain a type of skeptical practice. Sadly, those who are hooligans, that are nothing more than good con artists, will make it harder for those that do have a special ability to become recognized, or given any type of credibility.

Transformational Medicine

We are on a continuous path of transformation and self-healing. As our needs, and our lives change we find new forms of healing resonating stronger than other forms of healing. Providing a patient with what they need physically, mentally, and spiritually, is important.

Transformational medicine is a holistic medicine that uses natural therapies to help you regain your health and transform your life.

Your Mind - When we recognize the symptoms of our body there is almost always an underlying call for change and growth. Often we suppress our emotions and continue with our mindset, yet that mindset does not align with what it is we want in our lives.

Your Soul - When we release underlying blockages to our health it can lead to wellness, radiance, and vitality. Most will find they are experiencing feelings of joy and happiness, and their overall health improves.

Your Body - By addressing what is wrong with your body at the core and not just covering up symptoms you place yourself on a path to wellness again. For example, if you are a borderline diabetic rather than taking medication you might consider attacking the underlying cause, such as diet.

CHAPTER 12

THE ROLE OF FOOD

IN HEALTHY LIVING

You are what you eat, you eat too much, don't eat this, do eat that – the list of sayings and affirmations is endless.

From primeval times, mothers, doctors, health care givers, and a large array of good doers have made an arsenal of affirmations for what to eat that would fill more shelves than the library of congress.

Just look in any bookstore today and you will find shelf after shelf of diet books, self help health books that include suggestions on what to eat, and scientific books on many specific conditions that are based upon what we eat or do not eat.

So if we are what we eat, why don't we grow horns, smell like a pig, sprout wings or lettuce leaves and the like? If we eat too much, why is it that some who eat vastly more than others do not gain the same amount of weight?

If you are not supposed to eat candy to keep from getting diabetes, why is it that some people can have their daily chocolate bar, and munch on candy all day most of their lives and never gain a pound or get diabetes? Yet others can "just look at a box of candy and gain 5 pounds?

If I had a dollar for every list of things I should eat, my wealth would near that of Bill Gates. There are multitudes of suggestions of what to eat, and many appear to have rational reasons for the selections. In this book, we are not going to just suggest another list of dietary do's and don'ts. I have found that because each individual is physiologically different, the same suggestions just cannot apply to everyone, even if the desired 'end result' is the same. For example, weight loss.

Consequently, we've looked at conditions and methods of treating them. In part, this treatment will include suggestions of what to eat. But these suggestions will be tailored to various physiological parameters that are also covered throughout the book.

In the end, you will be able to match your desired results to a treatment plan that consists of medications, herbs, supplements, activity, and food. The food suggestions are part of an integral system of feeding not only the body, but also the mind and the spirit. In other words, in a manner appropriate for the new millennium, the whole person.

Good Fat Bad Fat

If you ask folks what food group they should avoid, most will probably answer "fats." While it's true that, in large amounts, some types of fat are bad for your health and your waist, there are some fats we simply can't live without.

The fats we must have include the omega-3 fatty acids, found in foods including certain fish, walnuts, and some fruits and vegetables. Omega-3s are considered "essential" fatty acids because the body can't make them and because without them, we literally can't survive.

"It not only plays a vital role in the health of the membrane of every cell in our body, it also helps protect us from a number of key health threats," says Laurie Tansman, MS, RD, CDN, a nutritionist at Mount Sinai Medical Center in New York.

Omega-3s have many health benefits including:

- ☑ A reduced risk of heart disease and stroke
- ☑ Assistance in reducing hypertension
- ☑ Assistance in reducing symptoms associated with depression
- ☑ Assistance in reducing symptoms associated with attention deficient disorder (ADD)
- ☑ Assistance in reducing symptoms associated with, joint pain and other rheumatoid problems, as well as certain skin ailments.
- ☑ Some research has even shown that omega-3s can boost the immune system and help protect us from an array of illnesses including Alzheimer's disease.

Just how do omega-3s perform so many health "miracles" in people? One way, experts say, is by encouraging the production of body chemicals that help control inflammation -- in the joints, the bloodstream, and the tissues.

They have another important job, and that is that they have the ability to reduce the negative impact of yet another essential type of fatty acid known as omega-6s. Found in foods such as eggs, poultry, cereals, vegetable oils, baked goods, and margarine, omega-6s are also considered essential.

Omega-6s also support skin health, lower cholesterol, and help make our blood "sticky" so it is able to clot. But, when omega-6s aren't balanced with sufficient amounts of omega-3s, problems can ensue.

"When blood is too 'sticky,' it promotes clot formation, and this can increase the risk of heart attack and stroke," says nutritionist Lona Sandon, RD, a spokeswoman for the American Dietetic Association. "But once you add omega-3s to the mix, the risk of heart problems goes down".

The latest research shows that the most promising health effects of essential fatty acids are achieved through a proper balance between omega-3s and omega-6s. The ratio to shoot for, experts say, is roughly 4 parts omega-3s to 1 part omega-6s. Read the supplement label to ensure that the ratios are appropriate.

Most of us, they say, come up dangerously short. "The typical American diet has a ratio of around 20 to 1 -- 20 omega-6's to 1 omega-3 -- and that spells trouble," says Sandon, an assistant professor of nutrition at University of Texas Southwestern Medical Center in Dallas.

While reducing your intake of omega-6s can help, getting more omega-3s from food is an even better way to go. Another concern is for those who take Omega supplements and unknowingly take a supplement containing more Omega 6's throwing the balance off even more.

How to Get What You Need

Omega-3 fatty acids are not one single nutrient, but a collection of several, including eicosapentaenoic acid (EPA) and docosahexaenoic acid (DHA). Both are found in greatest abundance in certain fish, and experts say that is one reason so many of us are deficient.

Over the past several years, the Food and Drug Administration and other groups have issued warnings about mercury and other harmful chemicals found in fish. This has caused many people to stop eating fish, which is a big mistake!

"People have taken the whole FDA advisory out of context including who it's for, which is primarily pregnant women, and small children," Tansman says. Moreover, Tansman says, even if you obey the FDA warnings in the strictest sense, the latest advisory says that up to 12 ounces of a variety of fish each week is safe for everyone. That's about half of what we need to get enough omega-3s.

"The omega-3s recommendation is two servings of fish a week," Tansman says. "At 3 to 4 ounces per serving, that's well below the FDA's safe limit of 12 ounces per week."

According to the American Heart Association, those looking to protect their hearts should eat a variety of types of fatty fish, such as salmon, tuna, and mackerel, at least twice a week. Those with heart disease should get 1 gram of omega-3s containing both EPA and DHA per day, preferably from fatty fish.

About 1.5 ounces of fish contain 1 gram of omega-3s. But even if you don't like fish (or choose not to eat it), you can still get what you need from dietary sources. Elaine Magee, MPH, RD, says one answer lies in plants rich in omega-3s - particularly flaxseed.

"It's safe to say this is the most potent plant source of omega-3," says Magee, author of The Flax Cookbook. While flaxseed contains no EPA or DHA, Magee says, it's a rich source of another omega-3 known as alpha-linolenic acid (ALA), which the body can use to make EPA and DHA.

Flaxseed is available in health food stores and many supermarkets, sold as whole seeds, ground seeds, or oil. Although flaxseed oil contains ALA, Magee says ground flaxseed is a much better choice because it also contains 3 grams of fiber per tablespoon, as well as healthy phytoestrogens. Other sources of omega-3s include canola oil, broccoli, cantaloupe, kidney beans, spinach, grape leaves, Chinese cabbage, cauliflower, and walnuts.

"About an ounce -- or one handful -- of walnuts have about 2.5 grams of omega-3s," says Sandon. "That's equal to about 3.5 ounces of salmon." Besides getting more omega-3s, you can also help your heart by replacing some omega-6s from cooking oils with a third fatty acid known as omega-9 (oleic acid). This is a monounsaturated fat found primarily in olive oil.

Though it is not considered "essential," the body can make some omega-9, by substituting it for oils rich in omega-6s; you can help restore the balance between omega-3s and omega-6s. In addition, you can gain some additional health benefits.

"Factors found in olive oil can also help boost the good cholesterol, which can also help your heart," says Magee.

It's important to ensure you are getting adequate good fat and avoiding bad fats to help your overall health.

Benefits of Unsaturated Fats

Eating monounsaturated and polyunsaturated fat lowers the risk of cardiovascular disease and interestingly, as I mentioned earlier in Chapter 5, it is said to also lower the incidence of gallstones.

As I have also shown in other parts of this book, unsaturated fats also lower the incidence of heart disease and its complications, whereas diets high in the saturated fats found in red meat and whole milk, promote the formation of gallstones and heart disease.

Water – Why We Need It

We all drink water on a regular basis usually to quench our thirst. Unfortunately, most people don't drink nearly enough water. Most people don't realize how important it is for the health of the body. Drinking water or failing to do so, affects every aspect of our bodies.

In reality, water ranks second only to oxygen as essential for life. We can go many days or even months without certain nutrients or minerals from food, but we can only survive a few days without water.

Water maintains our body temperature through perspiration. It is necessary to nourish the skin and to protect the joints and organs. The vital organs use water first, and the skin gets what is left over.

We have all seen pictures of people who are very dehydrated from being in the desert. When we stay well hydrated the skin will remain supple, and of course look younger and with less wrinkles.

Besides aiding in the necessary chemical processes in the body, water also aids in digestion, absorption, circulation, and various other functions such as maintaining the body temperature.

Drinking water can assist you in not gaining excess weight. When you don't drink enough water, your body secretes the hormone aldosterone, which causes tissues to hold on to various molecules including deposits of fat. Consequently, not drinking plenty of fresh water increases your body's fat deposits.

A recent study from the Harvard School of Public Health that studied 47,000 men over a 10-year period, indicated that those who drink sufficient water are 50% less likely to develop bladder cancer compared to those who drank just a glass of water per day. Most studies have shown that an adequate amount of water for the human body should be at least 3 liters per day.

Headaches can also be caused by not drinking sufficient water. Many people have been able to "cure" headaches by drinking 2-3 glasses of water when they feel a headache coming on.

Drinking water throughout the day helps keep your stomach feeling full and reduces the desire to eat. You may actually be thirsty rather than hungry when you get the urge to eat.

A study by the Fred Hutchinson Cancer Research Center in Seattle, Washington monitored women who drank more than 5 glasses of water a day and found that their risk of colon cancer was reduced by 45%.

Various studies have shown that even though relatively healthy individuals are not severely dehydrated, when they are mildly dehydrated on a chronic basis, their mental ability actually decreases.

Dr. Kleiner from the Institute of Physiology and Applied Sciences in Delhi noted that a 2% loss of body fluid affected short-term memory and reduced the ability to perform simple mathematical maneuvers.

We know that the amount of water inside of a cell can change within minutes. Muscles that are dehydrated by as little as 3% can cause a loss in a child's strength of about 10% as well as 12% loss in speed. This is obviously important to trained athletes, which is why we will often see a trained athlete drinking sufficient quantities of water.

Even if you are not a trained athlete, on average, you will lose 10 cups of water a day in a moderate temperature and only get back 4 of those from the food you eat. You will lose a cup and a half of water through your skin through perspiration; the kidneys will filter out 4 cups of water, and just breathing, will lose you one and a half cups of water per day.

So you see, the old adage about drinking 8 cups of water a day is really just a guideline. 8 cups is fine if those 8 cups are 8 ounce cups, and yet again this is still just a guideline.

If you are living in Phoenix Arizona, you need to add several cups of water for the ambient temperature. If you exercise, you need to add water for the loss that you will get from breathing heavily and perspiring. If you drink one cup of coffee you need to drink another 2 cups of water as coffee acts as a diuretic. Similarly, beer and other alcoholic beverages also act as diuretics.

Although you can often stop a headache with a quick glass of water, to fully rehydrate tired muscles that have gone without sufficient water it can take several hours to accomplish. The makeup of tissues which are predominantly water (skin, muscles, some connective tissue) take the longest time to recover from dehydration.

Water is extremely important for our bodies proper functioning, and although it is not as convenient to have to go to the bathroom every few hours to produce clear urine, it is a good sign that you are hydrating your body in a proper manner.

Unfortunately, as we get older, our bladders tend to be less cooperative at maintaining water for an extended period of time. It's even more important to drink more fluids as we get older. It just means that we have to be better at finding public restrooms when we are out of the house.

An interesting way of looking at mind body medicine is the way that Masaru Emoto does. His argument is that we start and maintain our life being nearly 90% water, in other words, we exist mostly as water.

His contention is that since water in a river is alive because it is moving and when water becomes stagnant it dies, the same is true about the water in our bodies. He goes on to indicate that this stagnation of water is because of the stagnation of one's emotions.

When you are living a full and enjoyable life, you feel better physically. If your life is filled with struggles and sorrow your body knows it (and it is reflected in your body-water composition). So when your emotions flow throughout your body, you feel a sense of joy and you move towards physical health.

This life force transports energy and needs to be kept clean. He argues that clean water makes beautiful crystals, and is an indication that all is well in the body. When there are problems, it is reflected in the water and the water is not as beneficial to the body.

Water is used in many therapies and weight loss programs. You will find this covered in the appropriate sections of the book. The bottom line is that we simply cannot live without water, just as we cannot live without air.

Preserving Skin

In the 21st century with a very large growing aging baby boomer population, concerns about how to stay young have become foremost in the minds of many. Aging is a natural process where certain aspects of the body deteriorate.

This is why we have a growing population with cardiovascular disease. The heart and blood vessels lose their elasticity and strain under the load of years of deposits laid down from the foods that we have eaten.

The pancreas also strains from having had to work hard all those years adjusting the blood sugar for all the sodas, and sweets that have been pushed thru its portals. When it finally gives up or fatigues, it gives the recipient adult onset diabetes.

The skin also goes thru an aging process. Since the skin is the mirror to the world, it is the one thing that we all notice in the aging individual. As we age, the skin cells divide more slowly. The padding just below the inner layer of skin (dermis) gets thinner. The supporting structures for the surface skin (elastin and collagen) loosen, and unravel, as we get older.

Consequently, the skin loses its elasticity and begins to sag and form furrows and wrinkles. Gravity has its expected effect on this process by pulling down the tissues even further.

Add to this, someone who has added excess adiposity, and the weight of that fat will pull the skin even further. Some people describe ageing as the formation of the pear shape in life: all the tissues gravitate to the middle.

Free Radicals

One reads about free radicals in many aspects of current medical literature. Very simply, when the body burns oxygen, it produces energy, and byproducts much like a combustion engine of a car. This process is called oxidation. Some of these byproducts that are produced are called oxidants. They can cause 'oxidative damage' to healthy cells of the body.

Let's take a look at a simple example: cut open an apple and leave it open to the air, it will soon become brown and oxidized. If you allow the apple to sit for several hours or days, it will go bad and get mushy.

The cells are releasing fluid to neutralize the oxidation. In some instances, the body will do the same thing. The body cells will turn brown (oxidize) and release fluid (edema) and eventually curl up and die.

Some scientists believe that most chronic, degenerative diseases are linked in some way to free radicals, and the damage they cause. If one were to extrapolate this theory, one could link diseases like arthritis, and diabetes to the formation of free radicals in the body. Because of the damage they invoke, heart disease and cancer are also considered potential side effects of the free radicals in the body.

There are several ways to combat this attack on the body. One of the most beneficial ways is by eating foods or supplements that are high in antioxidants. Leafy green vegetables and most fruits contain antioxidants. Vitamin C, E and Coenzyme Q10 are among the commonly used antioxidants.

Healing Foods

When I refer to healing foods, I am referring to foods that are good for all people to eat on a regular basis. Healing foods can help heal a vast variety of minor conditions and can often help specifically heal some more serious ones.

- ✓ What factors are considered if a food is to be listed as a 'healing food'?
- ✓ What is its impact on fats and their assimilation and deposition in blood vessels?
- ✓ What kind of fat does the food contain?

✓ Can it lower cholesterol levels?

✓ What is its influence on hormones and the intricate interdependence of hormones in the body?

✓ Does it contain any beneficial enzymes? Does it act to activate or assist any enzymes in carrying out any other essential body functions?

✓ Does it contain any substances that can help prevent various diseases, like cancer, diabetes, and heart disease?

✓ Does it contain any substances that can eliminate any particular toxins in the body?

✓ Does long-term use of the particular food contribute to any benefits to the person?

✓ Does long-term use provide anything more or less beneficial than short-term use?

8 Foods With Super Healing Powers

There are hundreds of extremely nutritious whole foods, but the dozen on this list do more than contribute healthy nutrients — they help you heal. In fact, every food listed here has multiple healing effects, from fighting cancer to reducing cholesterol, guarding against heart disease, and more.

Eat these super-healing picks and you will start feeling pretty super in no time at all. It is agreed upon by almost all, in every area of medicine, that these 8 foods truly are super foods.

1. Cherries

Cherries boast a huge amount of healing powers. Cherries pack a powerful nutritional punch for a relatively low calorie count. They're also packed with substances that help fight inflammation and cancer.

Lab studies have shown quercetin and ellagic acid, two compounds found in cherries, have been shown to inhibit the growth of tumors, and even cause cancer cells to commit suicide without causing any damage to healthy cells.

Cherries also have antiviral and antibacterial properties. Anthocyanin, another compound in cherries, is credited with lowering the uric acid levels in the blood, thereby reducing gout outbreaks, which are commonly caused by uric acid.

Researchers believe anthocyanins may also reduce your risk of colon cancer. Further, these compounds work like a natural form of ibuprofen, reducing inflammation and curbing pain. Regular consumption may help lower risk of heart attack and stroke.

In Chinese medicine, cherries are routinely used as a remedy for gout, arthritis, and rheumatism, as well as anemia, due to their high iron content.

2. Beans

Beans are a miracle food. They lower cholesterol, regulate blood sugar and insulin production, promote digestive health, and protect against cancer.

Beans offer fiber, protein, and antioxidants in a single food.

An assortment of phytochemicals found in beans has been shown to protect cells from cancerous activity by inhibiting cancer cells from reproducing, slowing tumor growth.

Researchers at the Harvard School of Public Health reported that women who consumed beans at least twice a week were 24% less likely to develop breast cancer, and multiple studies have tied beans to a reduced risk of heart disease, type 2 diabetes, high blood pressure, and breast and colon cancers.

Beans deliver a whopping amount of antioxidants, which help prevent and fight oxidative damage. In fact, the USDA's ranking of foods by antioxidant capacity places three varieties of beans (red beans, red kidney beans, and pinto beans) in the top four — and that's among all food groups.

Beans contain the amino acid tryptophan. Foods with high amounts of tryptophan can help regulate your appetite, aid in sleep, and improve your mood. Many are also rich in folate, which plays a significant role in heart health.

In Chinese medicine, various types of beans have been used to treat alcoholism, food poisoning, edema (particularly in the legs), high blood pressure, diarrhea, laryngitis, kidney stones, rheumatism, and dozens of other conditions.

Soybeans are an extremely versatile food. They are used to make a variety of food types from traditional tofu, to bean burgers, to very authentic tasting meat substitutes, to delicious desserts.

It's also important that we note that soybeans are a food that can easily fall into the category of healing foods. They contain a high percentage of fiber necessary in the treatment of many conditions.

They contain enzymes that destroy certain toxins. They contain isoflavones that are key to the above functions, and they are considered effective in lowering cholesterol and preventing some kinds of cancer.

Let's examine how one could incorporate this healing food into your diet without having to eat beans every day or the rather bland, plain tofu.

Tofu is the easiest manner of incorporating soybeans into your diet, because it is an incredibly versatile product. What is tofu? It is a white semisolid product made by taking the milk from the soybeans, and separating it into its components.

A curd is produced that is then pressed together. The resulting cheesy like substance is most commonly cut into blocks, and sold as the white tofu that one can find in most produce sections of grocery stores. It can be found fresh in the white state, soaking in its own whey (a thin, clear, light amber colored liquid) or in water. This is often how it is sold in Asian markets in big vats.

In western grocery stores, it is packaged in plastic containers with a preservative. It is also sold dried and flavored, such that it resembles jerky. The dried form can be reconstituted in a variety of dishes. Today, it is easy to find many baked forms in a number of flavors, as well as fermented forms, and aged forms. The aged forms look and taste a lot like the milk based dairy products but without cholesterol.

Tofu comes in several different textures that you can work with. The amount of whey pressed out of the soymilk curds during the production is what determines the texture. Soft tofu used commonly in Japan has a custard consistency, which is good for making dips, dressings, custards, puddings, and other desserts.

Firm tofu, of which there are several grades including one in which they add extra fiber has a medium density and is good for making scrambles and firmer desserts like cheesecake.

Extra-firm tofu is dense and holds its shape when sliced or cubed. The latter is best for making stir fried dishes, cutlets, and for marinating. You will find a great variety of readymade flavored tofu products now in most natural health stores.

Some of these are produced specifically for the 'fast food' industry, so that they can be eaten right out of the packet. There are also many products that can be used, instead of the dairy equivalent thus significantly reducing the fat content in one's diet.

By routinely using tofu-based products like tofu mayonnaise, sour cream, salad dressings, cheese, etc., you get the added benefit of the isoflavones from the tofu itself.

A few practicalities about tofu can be helpful to the cost-effective use of the product.

- ☑ Tofu is a product that can spoil just like any fresh food.
- ☑ Fresh tofu will keep better if you keep it in a glass or plastic container with a daily change of water.
- ☑ All tofu should be kept under refrigeration.
- ☑ For the baked and grilled tofu type products, just keeping them in airtight containers/bags in the refrigerator is appropriate.

If the only tofu that is available in your area is the Japanese style soft tofu, you can make it firmer for use in food preparations.

This is done by pressing out more of the whey. Slice the soft tofu into large slices, place it on a layer of absorbent towels, and cover it with a plate or breadboard. The more weight you apply and the longer you let it sit, the firmer it becomes. In 15 – 30 minutes tofu will usually firm up so that it can be used in cooking.

If you have more tofu than you can comfortably use during several days, drain the whey or water/preservative, wash the tofu in clear water, and wrap it in foil or heavy plastic then freeze it.

Some advise freezing it in the container with the liquid. If this is done, following the thawing process, the tofu must be washed/repeatedly soaked in fresh water.

Tofu frozen in this manner does get a very firm, crumbly texture, and can be used for scrambles or stir-fries very well. There are also a few varieties of vacuum-packed tofu that is stable at room temperature until it is opened.

3. Kiwi Fruit

This tiny, nutrient-dense fruit packs an amazing amount of Vitamin C. It's actually double the amount of Vitamin C found in oranges. They also have more fiber than apples, and they are even higher in potassium than bananas.

The unique blend of phytonutrients, vitamins, and minerals found in kiwi fruit helps protect against heart disease, stroke, cancer, and respiratory disease.

Kiwi fruit has natural blood-thinning properties, but without the side effects of aspirin. They also support vascular health by reducing the formation of spontaneous blood clots, reducing blood pressure, and lowering LDL cholesterol.

Multiple studies have shown that kiwi fruit not only reduces oxidative stress and damage to DNA but also prompts damaged cells to repair themselves.

4. Onions

Onions contain potent cancer-fighting enzymes, and antioxidants. Their consumption has shown to help reduce the risk of prostate and esophageal cancers, as well as having the potential to reduce mortality from coronary heart disease.

Research suggests that onions may help protect against stomach cancer. Onions contain sulfides that help lower blood pressure, and cholesterol, as well as a peptide that may help prevent bone loss by inhibiting the loss of calcium and other bone minerals.

Onions contain quercetin, which is a natural antihistamine that reduces airway inflammation, and helps relieve symptoms of allergies. Onions also boast high levels of Vitamin C, which are excellent for fighting colds and flu.

The anti-inflammatory properties of the onion help fight the pain and swelling associated with osteoarthritis, and rheumatoid arthritis. Onions are also extremely rich in sulfur, and they have antibiotic and antiviral properties, which help cleanse the arteries and slow/stop the growth of viruses, yeasts, and other disease-causing agents that can build up in an imbalanced diet. This makes onions an excellent choice for people who consume a diet high in protein, high in fat or sugar.

5. Carrots

Carrots are a great source of the potent antioxidants known as carotenoids. Diets high in carotenoids are linked to a decreased risk in postmenopausal breast cancer, bladder cancer, cervical cancer, prostate cancer, colon cancer, kidney cancer, ovarian cancer, and esophageal cancer.

Conversely, diets low in carotenoids have been associated with chronic disease, including heart disease and various cancers.

Research suggests that just one carrot per day could reduce your risk of lung cancer by half. The nutrients in carrots also reduce the occurrence of cardiovascular disease, stimulate the immune system, promote colon health, and support ear and eye health.

Carrots contain calcium, potassium, magnesium, phosphorus, fiber, Vitamin C, and an incredible amount of Vitamin A.

The alpha-carotene in carrots has shown promise in inhibiting tumor growth. Carrots also contain the carotenoids lutein and zeaxanthin, which work together to promote eye health and prevent macular degeneration and cataracts.

In Chinese medicine, carrots are claimed to treat rheumatism, kidney stones, tumors, indigestion, diarrhea, night blindness, ear infections, earaches, deafness, skin lesions, urinary tract infections, coughs, and constipation.

6. Cabbage

Cabbage is a powerhouse source of Vitamins K and C. Just one-cup supplies 91% of the recommended daily amount for Vitamin K, 50% of Vitamin C, fiber, and decent amounts of manganese, Vitamin B6, folate, and more. Best of all it's low in calories, and provides us with 11% more Vitamin C than oranges.

Cabbage contains high levels of antioxidant sulforaphanes that not only fight free radicals before they damage DNA, but also stimulate enzymes that detoxify carcinogens in the body.

Researchers believe this one–two approach may contribute to the apparent ability of cruciferous vegetables to reduce the risk of cancer more effectively than any other plant food group.

Numerous studies point to a strong association between diets high in cruciferous vegetables and a low incidence of lung, colon, breast, ovarian, and bladder cancers.

Cabbage minimizes allergic reactions, reduces inflammation, promotes gastrointestinal health, and builds strong bones. Cabbage is routinely juiced as a natural remedy for healing peptic ulcers due to its high glutamine content. It also provides significant cardiovascular benefit by preventing plaque formation in the blood vessels.

In Chinese medicine, cabbage is claimed to treat constipation, the common cold, whooping cough, depression and irritability, and stomach ulcers. When eaten, and used as a poultice, as a dual treatment, cabbage is helpful for healing bedsores, varicose veins, and arthritis.

7. Broccoli

It would be hard to find another single food with all of the health–promoting properties broccoli has. Just one cup of steamed broccoli provides more than 200% of the RDA for Vitamin C, nearly as much of Vitamin K, and roughly half of your daily allowance for Vitamin A.

It also contains B vitamins, fiber, iron, sulfur, and tons of other key nutrients. Calorie for calorie, broccoli contains about twice the amount of protein as steak plus it offers you all those protective phytonutrients.

Broccoli's phytochemicals fight cancer by neutralizing carcinogens, and accelerating their elimination from the body, in addition to inhibiting tumors caused by chemical carcinogens.

Studies show evidence that these substances help prevent lung and esophageal cancers and may play a role in lowering the risk of other cancers, including gastrointestinal cancer.

Phytonutrients called indoles found in broccoli help protect against prostate, gastric, skin, breast, and cervical cancers. Some research suggests that the reason that indoles may reduce the risk of prostate cancer is that they protect the structure of DNA.

Extensive studies have linked broccoli to a 20% reduction in heart disease risk. In Chinese medicine, broccoli is used to treat eye inflammation.

8. Kale

Kale is packed with powerful antioxidant, and anti-inflammatory qualities.

One cup of cooked kale contains an amazing 1,328% of the RDA for Vitamin K, 192% of the RDA for Vitamin A, and 89% of the RDA for Vitamin C. It's also a good source of calcium and iron.

Kale is in the same plant family as broccoli and cabbage, and, like its cruciferous cousins, it contains high levels of the cancer-fighting compound sulforaphane, by fighting free radicals in the body, thereby reducing the occurrence of gastric, prostate, breast, and skin cancers.

The indoles in kale have been shown to protect against breast, cervical, and colon cancers. The Vitamin K in kale helps build strong bones, and it promotes blood clotting, which protects the heart.

It also has more antioxidant power than spinach, protecting against free-radical damage. Kale is extra rich in beta-carotene, containing seven times as much beta-carotene as broccoli. It also contains lutein, and zeaxanthin, which is ten times more than what is found in broccoli. In Chinese medicine, kale is used to help ease congestion of the lungs.

You Are What You Eat - The Healthy Vegan Diet

Diseases such as diabetes, rampant obesity, coronary heart conditions, liver, and kidney failure, colon, and other cancers, to name but a few, are rising dramatically. What's more alarming, is that these diseases are affecting people at an increasingly young age. Of course, the fundamental cause is poor diet and nutrition.

One increasingly popular theory as to the reason for the epidemic of these conditions is based upon the fact that human beings are simply not "designed" to eat meat or dairy products. So, the human body either cannot process these "foods", or when the body does process them the result is a release of toxins.

Science has proven that most meat and dairy products are toxic to the human body in varying degrees, in some cases causing serious diseases that might not be immediately apparent.

For example, recently published research proves that eating bacon, or sausage increases the risk of contracting cancer by 6 times. Likewise, another published research result shows that eating steak has similar consequences.

In contrast, the current oldest person in the world is said to be a lady in Israel who is 120 years of age, and still does her own shopping, and her other chores on foot. She attributes her longevity, and activity to eating a proper diet of vegetables throughout her long life.

Other studies have proven that people eating a Vegan diet live on average 7 to 15 years longer than those eating animal and dairy products, which cannot be properly processed by the human body.

"The China Study" by Dr. T. Colin Campbell is based upon 20 years of intensive research of human diet involving many researchers based at three major universities in three countries. The results statistically show that the eating of animal products of any type has serious consequences for the body.

The conclusion is that natural plant based whole foods are by far and away the best and healthiest diet. Quite simply, the human body is designed to eat a plant-based diet.

I am not going to delve into the debate on evolution vs. intelligent design in this book, but it should be obvious from the facts that the primates from which humans evolved were, and still are, plant eaters. Accordingly, human physiology is designed to process plant material, and not animal flesh, which requires a completely different physiology.

Carnivores (cats, lions, dogs, eagles) all have very short digestive tracts (intestines) so that the food can go through the intestinal tract without absorbing all of the toxins from the other animal sources. Carnivores also have very sharp teeth to rip other flesh.

On the contrary, humans, other primates, horses, cows, etc. all have very long intestinal tracts. This is so that our kind can absorb all the nutrients from food that we are eating.

Cows of course have several stomachs to make sure that this process happens. When a human starts eating foods that contain things that we are not meant to eat or absorbed into the blood stream with our long intestinal tracts, the toxins, chemicals, and fat are absorbed and start causing damage.

Another major issue is how we are cooking our food. It makes sense not to want to boil, or heat foods to a high temperature, as it destroys most of the natural nutritional value of the food. Frying food not only heats the food to unnatural temperatures, but also converts originally healthy foods to very unhealthy ones.

We must remind ourselves that humans are, first and foremost, animals. How many other animals do we see in the wild eating microwaving or deep frying their food and consuming three or more supersized meals per day on a regular basis, and not getting any exercise? Furthermore, our idea of catching or gathering our meal is to drive to the grocery store or the drive-through.

Whole natural foods, eaten raw, baked or slightly steamed such as nuts, fruit, berries, grains, roots (potatoes & yams), etc. is our natural food, and gives us maximum nutrition.

 We should also keep in mind that food is first and foremost for nutrition. However, today most people eat for pleasure – to gratify the sense of taste. Such foods include fast food, highly modified 'gourmet' food, and pretty 'supermarket food'.

Supermarket food is laced with chemicals for preservation to increase shelf life, look pretty, and enhance taste, (i.e. MSG) with bright packaging carefully designed to lure the customer.

I remember speaking to a supermarket manager in England once who informed me that he had to make sure that the bananas had to be bright yellow, or else the ladies would not even look at them. To achieve this, he had to keep them in a chemical atmosphere right up until they were put out and 5 hours later they would develop a few black spots–so they would pull them, and use them for baking.

Our first priority for eating food should be for nutrition and sustenance. As Dr. Deepak Chopra says, "Cells function with the smallest possible expenditure of energy. Typically, a cell stores only 3 seconds of energy and oxygen inside its cell wall. It trusts totally on being provided for." Excessive consumption of food is not a necessity.

Taste should be considered to be a bonus, but is not vital in making something edible. This is one major factor in the development of disease in children, which can become debilitating when they grow older. Many children are given candy, sweet soda drinks, and of course fast food packed as "happy meals," and so on. There is nothing "happy" about obesity, diabetes, and other serious conditions. I was shocked to see a nurse giving her 1-year-old poutine (a French Canadian concoction of soggy French fries covered with cheese and high fat content gravy) as a treat! What will this child eat when he has some stress later in life?

A question that often arises is "if meat and dairy products are so risky, why do so many people eat them? The fact is, eating habits and choice of diet are very often family traditions that go back generations in the same way as religion and other family customs do.

Consequently, no one ever stops to consider whether parents are correct or not in the food choices they make for us as kids. Children simply assume from an early age that they must be.

The question every thinking person needs to ask is "what should I be eating"? There is no question when examining all the hard evidence, such as that presented in the book "The China Study", that the natural and therefore correct diet for all humans is natural, harvestable whole foods such as fruits, nuts, vegetables, grains, roots, fungi etc, eaten raw or slightly cooked.

It is no coincidence that all the largest and most powerful animals that ever lived eat exclusively plant foods. That's because plant foods contain the most energy, and nutrition to support their growth to their massive sizes (dinosaurs from the past and modern animals such as the elephant, rhinoceros and giraffe grow to such huge sizes and weight eating plant foods only). They can do this thanks to the phenomenal nutritional content in the plant foods they eat.

There are, of course, considerable ethical, not to mention karmic considerations that arise from supporting the appalling treatment of animals, birds and fish destined to become a meal on someone's table. Whether they are grown in appalling factory farms, or let to roam the wild open spaces, they are still living beings with a soul.

Animals are not objects placed here on earth for the convenience, or sometimes perceived inconvenience of humans. Rather, they are creatures created by a higher being just as we are, and therefore, should be treated as such.

Obviously there are many different beliefs in this realm. I hope this has provided you with "food for thought" and from a medical/scientific point-of-view will enable you to empower yourself, and family with a fresh, nutrient rich, natural diet.

The Truth About Eating Red Meat

Does eating red meat increase the risk of dying from heart disease or cancer? Fueled by research and high-profile campaigns by advocacy groups on both sides of the debate, it is a question that continually comes up. So let's set the record straight on what medical experts have to say.

1. Does eating red meat increase the risk of cancer and heart disease?

Some red meats are high in saturated fat, which raises blood cholesterol. High levels of LDL cholesterol are linked to an increased risk of heart disease. The answer isn't as clear when it comes to cancer. Many researchers believe red meat increases the risk of cancer, specifically colorectal cancer.

A recent National Institutes of Health-AARP study involving more than a half-million older Americans, concluded that people who ate the most red meat and processed meat over a 10-year-period were likely to die sooner than those who ate smaller amounts.

Those who ate about 4 ounces of red meat a day were more likely to die of cancer, or heart disease, compared to those who ate the least amount, about a half-ounce a day. As a result, epidemiologists classified the increased risk as "modest."

The meat industry contends that there is no link between red meat, processed meats, and cancer. They say that lean red meat fits into a heart-healthy diet yet have no scientific studies to back this up. Janet Riley, a senior vice president of the American Meat Institute, a trade group from the meat industry criticized the study.

As we have seen, many studies have found serious links. A large study followed more than 72,000 women for 18 years. It found that those who ate a Western-style diet, which was high in red meats, desserts, refined grains, and French fries, had an increased risk of heart disease, cancer, and death from other causes.

"The association between consumption of red and processed meats and cancer, particularly colorectal cancer, is very consistent," says Marji McCullough, PhD, a nutritional epidemiologist with the American Cancer Society.

In 2007, after a systemic review of scientific studies, an expert panel of the World Cancer Research Fund and the American Institute for Cancer Research concluded that "red or processed meats are convincing or probable sources of some cancers."

Their report says evidence is convincing for a link between red meat, processed meat, and colorectal cancer, and limited but suggestive for links to lung, esophageal, stomach, pancreatic, and endometrial cancers.

Rashmi Sinha, PhD, the lead author of the National Cancer Institute study, points to a large number of studies that link red meat consumption with chronic diseases. "The level of evidence is what people look at," Sinha says. "If there are 20 studies that say one thing and two studies that say the other thing, you believe the 20 studies."

2. If eating red meat does increase the risk of cancer, what's the cause?

To date, the cause is not clear, but there are several areas that researchers are studying, including:

- ✓ Saturated animal fat has been linked to breast cancer, and colon cancer, as well as to heart disease

- ✓ Carcinogens are formed when meat is cooked

- ✓ Heme iron, which is the type of iron found in meat, may produce compounds that can damage cells, leading to cancer

3. Are there any nutritional benefits from eating red meat?

Red meat is high in heme iron. Teenage girls and women in their childbearing years need iron. The body easily absorbs the heme iron in red meat, but iron can be obtained from many other sources.

Red meat also supplies Vitamin B12, which helps make DNA and keeps the nerve and red blood cells healthy; and zinc, which keeps the immune system working properly. Red meat provides protein, which helps build bones and muscles. As you move to a healthier lifestyle, all of these nutrients can be obtained from many plant sources as we have seen in this book.

4. Is pork a red meat or a white meat?

According to the U.S. Department of Agriculture, it is a red meat. The amount of myoglobin, a protein in meat that holds oxygen in the muscle, determines the color of meat. Pork is considered a red meat because it contains more myoglobin than chicken or fish.

5. Should I eat red meat?

Opinions differ on the amount of red meat a person may eat. However, most nutritionists suggest if you choose to eat red meat, you should focus on sensible small portion sizes and lean red meat cuts.

Alice Lichtenstein, DSc, professor of nutrition at the Human Nutrition Research Center on Aging at Tufts University, recommends asking yourself the following:

☑ Is red meat crowding out other important foods such as fruits, vegetables, and whole grains?

The American Institute for Cancer Research focuses on cancer prevention through diet, and physical activity and they advise avoiding all processed meats, such as sausage, deli meats, ham, bacon, hot dogs, and sausages, citing research that shows an increased risk of colon cancer.

6. Can grilling cause cancer?

High-temperature cooking of any muscle meat, including red meat, poultry, and fish can generate compounds called heterocyclic amines (HCAs) and polycyclic aromatic hydrocarbons (PAHs) in the food that may increase cancer risk.

7. How can you reduce potential cancer-causing compounds when grilling?

There are a number of steps that can help to prevent these compounds from forming or reduce your exposure to them. When grilling, be sure to choose low fat items. This will reduce the chance of grill flare-ups, which can deposit carcinogens on the food itself.

When grilling, avoid high heat; instead cook over medium heat or indirect heat. High heat can cause grill flare-ups and char food. You should also avoid frying, and broiling, which also subjects meat to high temperatures. Don't overcook meat. When meat is well done it contains more of the cancer-causing compounds. However, do make sure that meat is cooked to a safe internal temperature to kill bacteria that can cause food-borne illnesses. Reduce the amount of meat you grill. Rather than a steak, why not try a kabob that mixes meat and vegetables. Plant-based foods are not linked to HCAs. Always trim fat from the meat prior to cooking, and remove any charred pieces.

Meat Substitutes

Because of health concerns, or moral reasons, a great many people have given up eating meat. However, many still enjoy the texture of meat in their meals. Meat substitutes can be added to dishes to give substance and protein.

Most meat substitutes come from either soybean or wheat, but now there are also substitutes made from nuts, such as almond patties, and other grains like millet, quinoa, mushrooms, etc.

For many years, the Chinese have had a variety of meat substitutes. Many of these have wheat gluten as the base. I can remember a Buddhist monastery that I visited in China that served such meat substitutes, and many of the vegetarians in the group were concerned that the meal actually was not vegetarian.

Soy Products

Tofu

The humble soy bean has not only a great deal of a nutritive value which we will discuss in various other parts of the book but also a great variety of food forms that double as meat substitutes.

Soy products are a potent source of phytochemicals. They are low in saturated fat, contain essential fatty acids, are a good source of calcium, low in salt, and contain various vitamins and minerals including the B vitamins and iron.

Current studies have also shown that soy protein is beneficial to maintaining proper hormonal balance for females. Tofu is probably the most well known of soy products.

It was first used in China around 200 B.C. Tofu has long been a staple of Asian cuisine. In its natural form, tofu is a very bland food, which can be given to young children and sick adults as an easy form of protein and a soothing substance for upset stomachs. It contains all eight essential amino acids.

Tofu is available in many forms from a liquid yogurt like substance to the traditional pressed block that is cut and used in many types of cooking. In your local Asian store, you will find a vast variety of soy products.

The soy fibers can also be spun so that they can appear to be the same consistency as meat. Tofu is extremely versatile, and because it has little flavor of its own it easily soaks up the flavors of whatever it is cooked with.

There are two types of tofu that you'll want to try: the first is fresh, water packed tofu, which must always be refrigerated. The firmer forms of tofu can be cooked, sliced in stir-fries, or mashed for eggless scrambled eggs. Tofu can be used as a filling in sandwiches cubed in casseroles and made into burgers.

The softer form of tofu can be creamy and used in desserts and also in savory dishes. Textured vegetable protein (TVP), a soy product, is available as a mince or chunks. It can be flavored or unflavored and has a very long shelf life. It is easily prepared just by adding water, letting it stand and then cooking it in whatever dish is desired.

The second type is silken tofu, which is packed in aseptic boxes, and usually not refrigerated. Silken tofu is used for making a chocolate cream pie but will fall apart if you try to make it into shish kebab. When baking tofu, cook it in a marinade so it will soak up more flavors.

To give tofu a meatier texture, try freezing it for 2 to 24 hours and then defrosting it. Pressing the water out of it under blocks/weight is another way of changing its texture.

Tempeh

Tempeh is a traditional Indonesian food and is made from fermented soybeans and other grains. In its final form it has a chewy texture that can be steamed, baked, or fried. Tempeh is very high in protein and a variety of minerals and vitamins.

Unlike tofu (which is bland and absorbs any flavor you give it) and is made from soybean milk, tempeh contains whole soybeans, which makes it much denser and has a very distinctive flavor. Because of tempeh's density, it should be marinated in a strong flavorful liquid for at least one hour prior to cooking. This will also soften it up and make the flavor mellower.

Wheat Gluten (Seitan)

Seitan, which is also known as wheat gluten, is derived from wheat and it is an excellent source of protein. This product is available in many forms, and it comes flavored or unflavored. The common varieties that are seen in most Asian grocery stores include mock duck, pseudo chicken, pseudo turkey, beef chunks, pseudo abalone and a variety of curries.

Whole Grains and Legumes

Whole grains are an excellent source of protein, fiber, B vitamins, and zinc. Legumes include navy beans, pinto beans, garbanzo beans, kidney beans, peanuts, lentils, split peas, and black-eyed peas. Use beans as a protein source in salads, soups, stews, veggie patties, and rice dishes.

Nuts and Seeds

Nuts and seeds are another good source of protein. Although some are high in 'good' fats, they can be used in many recipes as a meat substitute, and are still lower in 'bad' fat than most animal protein.

Nuts and Their Nutritive Values

Nuts have long had a bad rap for being high in fat and calories, prompting weight-conscious people to relegate nuts to their lists of forbidden foods. But as researchers take a closer look at walnuts, almonds, and other nuts, they're discovering these delicious, crunchy foods are packed with vitamins, minerals, and antioxidants. And that fat we were so wary of? Turns out it's good for our hearts. That was the conclusion of the Food and Drug Administration (FDA), which released a qualified health claim that states eating 1.5 ounces (about a handful) of nuts a day may reduce the risk of heart disease.

That's because most of the fat in nuts is monounsaturated and polyunsaturated, which have been shown to lower levels of LDL ("bad" cholesterol). These fats are important because they have an anti-inflammatory effect on the body and can help repair tiny muscle injuries that create inflammation.

Not just any nut will do, however. The FDA includes six nuts in its qualified health claim, but a few others didn't make the cut, including Brazils, macadamias, and cashews. These nuts have relatively high levels of saturated fat, which over time can clog arteries, and lead to heart disease.

It's also a good idea to steer clear of prepackaged nut mixes, which are often coated in oils and salt. Instead, buy the following types of nuts raw and toast them in the oven or on the stovetop to bring out their full, rich flavor.

Almonds

Why: A recent study found that the fiber in almonds actually blocks some of the nut fat from being digested and absorbed; participants also reported feeling satisfied after eating almonds, so they naturally compensated for the calories in the nuts by eating less during the day.

One serving of almonds provides 35% of the Daily Value (DV) for Vitamin E.

How: Add almonds to your breakfast cereal or yogurt. Mix into salad.

One Ounce = 23 nuts 163 calories, 6 g protein, 14 g fat

Peanuts

Why: Peanuts are technically not nuts — they're legumes and belong to the same family as beans and peas. They have a low glycemic index, which means they are digested slowly, and help maintain a balanced blood-sugar level.

Peanuts also contain resveratrol, the same phytochemicals found in red wine are thought to protect against heart disease.

How: Use peanut butter as a sauce base for a Thai noodle dish or lightly brown peanuts in a skillet and add them to other dishes.

Caution: Read the label of packaged or bottled peanut butter. Many of the commercially available brands have sugar, and hydrogenated oil as a main ingredient. These may have an overall lower fat content because they do not contain many peanuts; only buy the product that says peanuts and salt as the ingredients.

One Ounce = 28 nuts 166 calories, 7 g protein, 14 g fat

Walnuts

Why: Walnuts are very rich in the plant-based omega-3 fatty acid ALA, which decreases inflammation that can damage arteries, and may help reduce the breakdown of bone.

Studies have also shown that walnuts can increase levels of HDL (good cholesterol) while lowering LDL (bad cholesterol).

How: Add walnut oil to salad dressing or use crushed walnuts to make a pesto sauce. Chop walnuts and mix into tacos for added crunch.

One Ounce = 14 halves 185 calories, 4 g protein, 19 g fat

Pistachios

Why: These tasty, little green nuts are high in lutein, an antioxidant typically found in dark leafy vegetables that's been shown to protect our eyes from macular degeneration.

In one recent study, participants who ate 1.5 ounces of pistachios every day lowered their total cholesterol levels, while participants who ate three ounces a day saw an even more dramatic drop.

How: Sprinkle pistachios on salads. Add crushed or pulverized pistachios to meat loaf in place of the beef.

One Ounce = 49 pistachios 158 calories, 6 g protein, 13 g fat

Pecans

Why: One study ranked the antioxidant capacity of 100 different foods and found that pecans are one of the top 15 sources of antioxidants.

In another study, pecan antioxidants were shown to prevent LDL from building up in arteries and lowered total cholesterol levels.

Compared with other nuts, pecans have one of the highest levels of phytosterols, a group of plant chemicals that may help protect against cardiovascular disease.

How: Add pecans to pancake batter, or coarsely chop and toss with pasta. Mix finely chopped or pulverized pecans into 'meatless' loaf or patties.

One ounce = 19 halves 196 calories, 3 g protein, and 20 g fat

Hazelnuts

Why: Hazelnuts have the highest nut level of folate, a B vitamin. Research indicates that it, along with other B vitamins, may also lower the risk of heart disease, cancer, and depression.

Hazelnuts contain moderate levels of potassium, calcium, and magnesium, all of which can help lower blood pressure.

How: Add roasted hazelnuts to asparagus with lemon vinaigrette. They also go well with things like granola.

One Ounce = 21 nuts 178 calories, 4 g protein, 17 g fat
The following nuts unfortunately have high fat content, so eat these nuts with saturated fat sparingly.

Brazil Nuts

One Ounce: 6 nuts, 186 calories, 4 g protein, 19 g total fat

The Bad News: 4 g saturated fat per one-ounce serving

The Good News: Highest amount of selenium of any food; this mineral helps eliminate free radicals that can lead to cancer.

Macadamia Nuts

One Ounce: 11 nuts, 204 calories, 2 g protein, 21 g total fat

The Bad News: 3 g saturated fat, and more calories than any other nut

The Good News: High in thiamine, a type of B vitamin that helps metabolize carbohydrates into energy.

Cashew Nuts

One Ounce: 18 nuts, 157 calories, 5 g protein, 12 g total fat

The Bad News: 2.5 g saturated fat per one-ounce serving

The Good News: Rich in copper and magnesium as well as zinc, which is important for a healthy immune system.

Net Carbs and Artificial Sweeteners

When is a carb not a carb? That's the question many carb-conscious dieters are facing, as they struggle to keep their carb counts within the strict limits recommended by low-carb diets.

In an effort to cash in on the low-carb craze, food manufacturers have invented a new category of carbohydrates known as "net carbs," which promises to let dieters eat the sweet and creamy foods they crave without suffering the carb consequences.

But the problem is that there is no legal definition of the "net," "active," or "impact" carbs popping up on food labels, and advertisements. The only carbohydrate information regulated by the FDA is provided in the Nutrition Facts label, which lists total carbohydrates and breaks them down into dietary fiber and sugars. The FDA has not evaluated information or claims about carbohydrate content that appear outside that box.

"These terms have been made up by food companies," says Wahida Karmally, DrPH, RD, and Director of Nutrition at the Irving Center for Clinical Research at Columbia University. "It's a way for the manufacturers of these products to draw attention to them and make them look appealing by saying, 'Look, you can eat all these carbs, but you're really not impacting your health, so to speak.'"

Although the number of products touting "net carbs" continues to grow, nutrition experts say the science behind these claims is fuzzy, and it's unclear whether counting net carbs will help or hurt weight loss efforts.

What's in a Net Carb?

The concept of net carbs is based on the principle that not all carbohydrates affect the body in the same manner. This is hogwash.

Some carbohydrates, like simple or refined starches and sugars, are absorbed rapidly and have a high glycemic index, meaning they cause blood sugar levels to quickly rise after eating. Excess simple carbohydrates are stored in the body as fat. For example, white bread, white rice, and sweets.

Other carbohydrates, such as the fiber, found in whole grains, fruits, and vegetables, move slowly through the digestive system, and much of it isn't digested at all, which is called insoluble fiber. This is what you want.

Also, in this category of largely indigestible carbohydrates are sugar alcohols, such as mannitol, sorbitol, xylitol, and other polyols, which are modified alcohol molecules that resemble sugar. These substances are commonly used as artificial sweeteners.

In calculating net carbs, most manufacturers take the total number of carbohydrates a product contains, and subtract fiber and sugar alcohols, because these types of carbohydrates are thought to have a minimal impact on blood sugar levels.

For example, the label on a Power Bar's new double chocolate flavor "Protein Plus Carb Select" bar says it has "2 grams of impact carbohydrates." The Nutrition Facts label on the product says it has 30 grams of total carbohydrates. Just below the nutrition facts box, the "impact carb facts" box provided by the manufacturer explains:

"Fiber and sugar alcohols have a minimal effect on blood sugar. For those watching their carb intake, count 2 grams." That's 30 grams minus the bar's 27 grams of sugar alcohols and 1 gram of fiber.

The Skinny on Sugar Alcohols

Researchers say the impact of sugar alcohols on blood sugar levels and the body is not fully understood and they may also cause problems in some people.

"There are some sugar alcohols that can raise your blood sugar," says Karmally. "Certain sugar alcohols do have a higher glycemic index, and they still are not counted as carbohydrates by these companies."

"When you tell a person 'net carbs' or 'impact carbs,' it's very confusing," says Karmally. "A person with diabetes may think, 'It's fine for me to have as much as I want.'"

People with diabetes are advised to closely monitor their intake of carbohydrates because their bodies can't produce enough insulin to keep blood sugar levels within a safe range.

"I think we should not misguide people, and make them aware that these sugar alcohols also contribute calories," says Karmally. "Too much of them can actually have a bad effect, and some of them can also have a laxative effect."

Although sugar alcohols have been used in small amounts in items like chewing gums for years, researchers say little is known about the long-term effects of consuming large amounts of these substances.

When considering carbohydrates, you should also focus on calories. Foods that have calories have an impact on weight management, because of the number of calories you consume.

The old adage of *calories in must equal calories out* needs to be followed in order to control weight. As we have said, in many ways in this book, eating foods that are naturally low in refined carbohydrates, such as fruits and vegetables, rather than highly processed foods like snack bars, pastas, and sweets, is the way to go. Whole foods, like whole grains, fruits, and vegetables, should be the foundation of your diet.

Positive Nutrition

We've been talking about food - what's good for you, what's not, super foods, food fats and bad fats, and more. Now let's cover here what some of the most important changes are that we must all make to improve the quality of our nutrition.

Even after public campaigns regarding the benefits of eating lots of fruits and vegetables, the average consumption still is only around 2.5 portions per day.

Dietary nutritional deficiencies are a critical problem in our society. It is almost impossible to obtain all the micronutrients we need if we eat the standard modern day diet of 2000 cal.

Over the past few decades, unfortunately, too many Americans and Canadians have let themselves go. This has resulted in a frightening increase in obesity and obesity related illness such as heart disease, diabetes, stroke, and joint problems.

It's not totally unreasonable to understand how this happens, when you look at all types convenience foods, and the overall lack of exercise of this computer age generation. Nutrition should be at the top of our public health and families' personal agenda.

It is important that we start eating the right things from a very early age. At the age of six months a variety of foods can be introduced into your child's diet. In fact, failure to do so will result in a child who as an adult refuses the foods that are known to be healthy for our diet on a long-term basis.

For example, the child who has only been on a diet of sweetened juices, milk, sugared cereals, bland pasta, and ground up baby foods, will learn to refuse food, or he/she will become addicted to a typical American diet when he/she is older.

Research in the United Kingdom has shown that the average school-age children actually prefer junk food. This is totally unlike similar research in children in Greece, Italy, and Egypt. It just validates that we have developed a generation in love with junk food.

Children's menu should be a balanced diet with a mixture of protein, carbohydrates, and healthy fats. We will talk about various modifications of the traditional balanced diet in later chapter. An excess of only one type of food at the expense of the rest of a basic diet is undesirable.

One's diet should also be rich in trace elements and vitamins. Unfortunately, the vitamin content of the foods we eat is falling for many reasons including modern farming, and marketing practices, which result in food that is not fresh by the time it reaches the supermarket shelves. Research also indicates that this delay can result in the vitamin content being depleted.

Most traditional nutritionists try to maintain a balanced diet and many have taken it further, demonstrating that this fat content should have only a very small percent of saturated fat.

If one listens to some of the newer philosophies regarding the glycemic index, and carbohydrates, the higher the index the faster these foods are absorbed from the gastrointestinal tract in to the metabolic system.

Carbohydrates with a low glycemic index are nutritionally the best. As much of the carbohydrate as possible should be complex polysaccharides because these take much longer to digest in our gastrointestinal tract. Examples of this include whole-grains, baked potatoes, etc. These are preferred over highly refined white bread or sugary sweets, which of course, are also carbohydrates.

Vegetable protein is definitely the preferred protein. This is the protein found in beans, tofu, legumes, peas, nuts, etc. Certain kinds of animal protein can also be added to the diet. There are good fats and bad fats. Omega-3, 6, & 9 essential fatty acids are found in various sea vegetables like algae, flaxseed, and various oily fish like salmon and sardines.

Having a sufficient quantity of the essential fatty acids found in omega-3 and 6 will benefit the health of your heart. It is also been found that the omega-3 fatty acids also benefit the brain, especially in childhood. In fact, it has been shown that mothers who consume omega-3s while pregnant will have children that have higher brain function in early infancy.

As of yet, there have been no long-term studies on this but this added advantage of brain function likely goes far beyond those childhood years and may reduce the incidence of Alzheimer's disease, and other dementias.

Besides consuming the appropriate amount of the right fats, protein, and carbohydrates, we also need to ensure that sufficient amounts of fiber are also in the diet. If you consume large quantities of fruits and vegetables you will consume sufficient fiber and provide your body with essential vitamins and trace minerals.

The old saying of five different fruits and vegetables during the day still holds today, as does eating foods of a variety of colors. Variety in one's diet may not only be the spice of life, it may be just what's needed to preserve life.

In our go-go-go life, one often says "I don't have the time to eat five portions of fruit and vegetables during the day, with my busy life." A few of those portions may be in the form of fruit smoothies, dried fruit, and frozen vegetables. Fresh salads are important on a regular basis, and they should be made out of a variety of vegetables, not just iceberg lettuce.

Because a great number of the foods we eat do not contain all the nutrients that we need as a result of being grown on deficient soil, it is important that you also take vitamins and/or other food supplements along with the foods you eat. Only then can you be sure of receiving adequate vitamins and minerals.

CHAPTER 13

HERBS, VITAMINS & SUPPLEMENTS

Herbs and vitamins can replace missing nutrients in foods, or they can be used in larger quantities to affect a response in a certain body system or part-like using Hawthorne as a heart tonic. Various amino acids such as inositol and methionine can facilitate certain herbs.

Nutritional Supplementation Against Stress

Stress causes an increase in utilization of certain nutrients in the body. Nutrition will affect the composition of every person's chemical composition. Stress burns up protein by eliminating some of the essential amino acids.

B Vitamins

When the body is under stress, your body needs extra B vitamins: B1-thiamine, B2-riboflavin, B3-niacin, B6-pyridoxine, B5-pantothenic acid, biotin, para-amino-benzoic acid (PABA), choline, Inositol, and folic acid.

B vitamins are not stored in the body and must be supplied in sufficient quantities through the diet. This is especially true during times of stress. All B vitamins are water-soluble and are excreted through the urine. Alcohol consumption also increases the need for more B vitamins, as they are required to burn off the excess alcohol in the body.

Vitamin C

Stress burns up vitamin C. Smoking also burns up vitamin C. According to Doctor Linus Pauling, one cigarette burns up 50 milligrams of vitamin C, and shortens your life expectancy by fifteen minutes. As we already know, vitamin C fights free radicals diminishing the structural changes, and cell mutations that occur when the iron poor molecules steal ions from healthy cell molecules.

Good Oils

Stress created by cardiac orientated problems such as high cholesterol and triglycerides can be elevated by l-carnitine. Oils rich in essential fatty acids such as linseed oil and fish oil are also beneficial in alleviating this stress.

Calcium & Magnesium

These minerals are plentiful in the body and are needed for metabolism and muscle/nerve function. Magnesium is particularly beneficial to the heart.

Zinc

It has been shown that men with benign prostatic hypertrophy have low levels of zinc in their prostatic fluids, and supplementation with zinc may reduce the enlargement. The prostate tends to contain a higher concentration of zinc than any other organ in the body. Therefore, a zinc supplement has been shown to benefit some men.

Selenium

Studies have shown selenium added to the diet can inhibit the growth of the prostate particularly growth from cadmium. Adequate doses range from 100 to 200 mcg daily.

L-Carnitine

This well-known amino acid is used in weight reduction/fat loss. The body stores fat as an additional energy supply in times of high activity and need. If one doesn't exercise extensively, and burn off calories, the excess fat that is consumed then turns into stored fats. When we exercise there will be an initial carbohydrate fuel burn.

GABA

Gamma-aminobutyric acid (GABA) is an amino acid that is useful in stress and anxiety. GABA acts at the same receptor sites as Valium and other allopathic anti anxiety agents. GABA will fill the receptor sites and prevent anxiety related messages from being sent to the brain's motor neuron centers.

GABA actually lowers the excitatory level of the cell that's about to receive this incoming message. When there is prolonged stress supplementation with GABA, Inositol and Niacinamide can affect anxiety moderation much as other tranquilizers.

Amino Acid Tyrosine or Phenylalanine

Certain studies have shown that various mood disorders can be controlled with the amino acid Tyrosine or Phenylalanine. In 1980, research at Harvard Medical School determined that a lack of available Tyrosine resulted in a deficiency of Norepinephrine, and that this deficiency in the brain was related to various mood problems. Certain allopathic anti-depressants actually attempt to increase the Norepinephrine levels much as supplementation with l-tyrosine would.

Useful Healing Herbs

Cat's Claw (Una De Gato)

Cat's Claw is the potent red inner bark and the root of this tropical plant and has a variety of uses. Its uses are generated usually from the overall enhancement of the immune system, its anti-inflammatory, anti-oxidant and anti-viral uses.

In all the studies that have been done, Cat's Claw has been shown to be safe, and generally well tolerated. There are certain individuals who find it irritating to the gastrointestinal tract. This is interesting because it can also help the gastrointestinal tract with benefit to the mucus lining of the intestines.

Its main use is as an anti-inflammatory, decreasing pain and inflammation of arthritis and other inflammatory conditions, such as peripheral edema (swelling), and irregular cycles seen in women with premenstrual syndrome.

This herb has been shown to reduce allergic reactions in people with asthma, again most probably due to healing of mucus membranes in the lining of the lungs. Cat's claw has been shown to inhibit platelet aggregation and consequently thrombosis.

Cat's Claw is high in anti oxidants including beta carotene and has traditionally been used as a tonic in Indian cultures. This is most likely due to its effect on the immune system increasing the defensive activity of various immune cells such as phagocytes or lymphocytes. Similarly, it has been utilized in fatigue reducing the effects of stress. Cat's Claw is generally used in doses of 2 to 6 grams a day in either capsules or tea.

Saw Palmetto (Serenoa Repines)

Saw Palmetto berries are found on this small palm tree native to Southeastern United States, which has been used by Native American Indians for many centuries.

It is repudiated to be an aphrodisiac and has been used as such in Western Europe for many centuries. Although the aphrodisiac qualities have never been proven there are a number of controlled studies that have shown that Saw Palmetto can help in benign prostatic hypertrophy (BHP).

Benign prostatic hypertrophy often happens to men in the middle age. The prostate begins to grow interfering with urinary flow and causing uncomfortable pressure in the bladder. Some researchers believe that excessive amounts of testosterone in the prostate cause enlargement, while others point to decreases in the production of estrogen, with the most popular current belief that it has something to do with testosterone levels.

The prostate is part muscle & part gland and normally about the size of a walnut. It lies just below the bladder and surrounds a segment of the urethra, the tube through which urine and semen exit the body. The prostate contributes most of the fluid that comprises semen, which carries the sperm when it is ejaculated. When a man has BHP, it can make urination very painful and slow.

Since it affects nearly half of all men over 40 and 75% of those over the age of 60, it is important that it is treated. It can be surgically corrected, and there are certain allopathic medications such as finasteride, which have been known to also help.

The more than 20 double blind placebo controlled clinical studies on Saw Palmetto, seems to show it reduces inflammation and fluid accumulation in the prostate and inhibits the conversion of testosterone to dihydrotestosterone.

Pygeum

This is another herb that is helpful for men with prostatic or libido problems. It apparently works by reducing inflammation and fluid retention in the prostate and repairs damage to blood vessels.

It also lowers some cholesterol. This has been used in France and Italy for some years. Plant sterols have beneficial effect on the prostate and are commonly derived from pumpkin seeds, saw palmetto and Pygeum.

Phytoestrogens

Vegetarians are shown to have lower instance of prostate enlargement and a lower mortality from prostate cancer. It is thought that this is due to relatively high levels of phytoestrogens in the diet notably soy products, legumes, whole grains, sprouts, linseed, and other vegetables.

Other studies have shown similar results with additions of vitamin E, selenium, zinc, evening primrose and essential fatty acids. And lastly, it is known that high fat and alcohol content in the diet tends to aggravate prostate problems.

Tumeric Extract (Curcumin)

Curcumin is the active ingredient in turmeric and is used in many Ayurvedic and other herbal combinations. It has significant anti-inflammatory activity and is a powerful antioxidant.

Flavonoids-Anthocyanidins

Flavonoids are another important aspect of the inflammatory process and various other processes in the body. The term flavonoids refers to a generic term embracing a particular type of plant pigment that is found in many kinds of fruits, vegetables, nuts, seeds and various other parts of plants. They form a widely distributed group of secondary plant products that are ingested with a healthy diet.

These phytonutrients are useful in conditions where vascular fragility and increased cellular permeability occur. By assisting in maintaining membrane integrity and function and by also protecting the enzyme and chemical processes necessary to have DNA function; the flavonoids achieve this by not allowing oxidation of lipid, proteins, and nucleic acids.

These oxidative reactions have been implicated in the development in numerous diseases for instance Atherosclerosis. Flavonoids are active in hydrophilic and lipophilic systems, working equally well in water as well as fat (lipid) environment.

This makes them unique as antioxidants. They are, therefore, classified as non essential anti oxidants even though they can function much like the antioxidant enzymes and nutritive anti oxidants such as vitamin E, beta-carotene, vitamin C and Selenium.

Flavonoids are able to inhibit arachidonic acid released from membrane sites and its subsequent conversion to inflammatory metabolites. Arachidonic acid breaks down to potentially harmful metabolites, which are inflammatory in nature and can aggravate or precipitate cardiovascular or arthritic pains.

The blocking done by the flavonoids is also done by aspirin and non-steroidal anti-inflammatory medications (NSAIDS - like Celebrex, Advil, Motrin, etc). The latter two are commonly used for treatment of arthritis and pain.

Flavonoids are used in a natural way of helping with cardiovascular disease. Quercetin is a type of flavonoid that is said to inhibit the oxidation of low-density lipoproteins LDL, "bad" cholesterol. Flavonoids also inhibit cyclooxygenase, which leads to lower aggregation of platelets (thinner blood), and a reduction in the possibility of blood clots occurring. A recent study by Hertzog in Holland showed that flavonoid intake was inversely related to mortality from coronary heart disease at a significant level.

The researchers had calculated the dietary antioxidant flavonoids in the Dutch diet. To eliminate confounding variables, a multivariate regression approach was used to adjust the relative risk values for various substances in the diet.

The effect of flavonoid intake on the age-adjusted mortality from coronary heart disease became even more significant after adjusting for the dietary confounding variables. In other words, consuming flavonoids was beneficial for the heart and the rest of the cardiovascular system.

In inflammatory joint disease, it is postulated that a combination of the suppression of inflammatory prostaglandin synthesis and the stimulation of collagen cross-linking (proline hydroxylation) may be the responsible mechanism.

Proanthocyanidin flavonoids are known to affect collagen integrity. They apparently cross link collagen fibers, which results in the reinforcement of the natural cross linking this protein collagen matrix of all connective tissue in the human body. By doing this, they can help reduce symptoms of varicose veins, and other capillary fragility conditions such as easily bruising.

As with many foods, we're finding new therapeutic effects that some plant foods have. The phytochemicals can be present in large quantities. These are helpful in guarding the body against disease. We have long known that fruits and vegetables are helpful against chronic disease.

This appears to be because of the non-nutrients such as the flavonoids, the anti oxidants and the collagen stabilizing properties of these in addition to the high density of micronutrients.

Carotenoids

Carotenoids are found widely in fruits and vegetables. Carotenoids include alpha and beta-carotene, vitamin A, lycopene, lutein, zeaxanthin etc. Carotenoids are a strong antioxidant and consume free radicals in the body.

They are found in various foods especially in pigmented plants (those with lots of color). Studies by the U.S Department of Agriculture, Harvard University have shown some of the benefits of the carotenoids.

No absolute proof has been shown, but there is good evidence that macular degeneration, which is the degeneration of the back of the retina of the eye, may be prevented with dietary carotenoids. This prevention has been extended to anti oxidants such as vitamin C and E, and also lutein, lycopene, and zeaxanthin, which are found in the eye.

The exact function is unknown, but these colored pigments may be functioning as filters against certain wavelengths of light. It may also be that carotenoids actually increase the density of the macular pigments and thereby protect the retina from macular degeneration. Statistically, people who eat more carotenoids, like carrots, in their diet have less cataracts and age related macular degeneration.

Isoflavones

Isoflavones from soybeans are powerful antioxidants. Daidzein and genistein are two of these that are also useful as we noted in cardiovascular health maintenance.

Phosphatidylserine

Phosphatidylserine is a phospholipid that is felt to maintain proper brain chemistry and mental function.

Tocotrienolos

Tocotrienolos are powerful antioxidants said to be even more powerful than Tocopherols of the vitamin E family.

N-acetylcysteine

N-acetylcysteine - this amino acid derivative increases the antioxidant Glutathione.

Quercetin

Quercetin as is a bioflavonoid with strong anti-inflammatory, and antioxidant capacities. It is said to inhibit histamine production, and to reduce leukotrienes, which are inflammatory substances.

Polyphenol Flavonoids

Polyphenol Flavonoids are potent anti oxidants used to maintain connective tissue integrity in the skin, blood vessels, etc. These are generally from pine bark, grape seeds, and green tea extracts.

Alpha Lipoic Acid

Alpha Lipoic Acid is an antioxidant and detoxifying agent, which is necessary for proper nerve cell growth. It is also known to protect carotenoids in tissues.

Flower Remedies

Flower remedies are popular in the British Isles. They are said to act as mood altering agents. There are no scientifically acceptable studies that have shown to prove the claims made for these substances, but there is a large group of followers that feel that flower essences are a reliable treatment for a host of emotional difficulties.

They show no side effect, and if they can be substituted for potent psychiatric drugs, they are certainly a useful addition to an armamentarium of natural healing. The theory goes that when you drink just several drops of a flower essence, the flower's energy vibrates through your body, making your energy and you "more harmonious".

This theory goes on to state that you are balancing your energy by taking the flower essences, which will allow you to overcome emotional problems, resetting the body's cells to their correct vibration frequency. The flower essences are so diluted that it is unlikely that there are any biochemical changes, which actually occur with their use similar to homeopathic remedies.

An interesting use of Bach Rescue Remedy is the dog community. Many have used Rescue Remedy to calm a nervous or anxious dog, before a veterinary appointment, when placed in a new home, during a summer storm, and a host of other situations.

What's fascinating is that around 90% of the dogs given the remedies become more relaxed within minutes. Dogs have no way of knowing so they present an interesting, yet unscientifically provable, testing of flower remedies.

SAM-e (S-Adenosyl Methionine)

This is an amino acid derivative that has shown to benefit brain, joint, and liver function. Methionine is an essential amino acid that is activated by the reaction of ATP (adenosine triphosphate) to form SAM-e.

The liver is an organ that filters the blood and manufactures various elements in the body. The synthesis of glutathione and the enzymes: glutathione peroxidase and glutathione-S-transferase; are supported by SAM-e.

Glutathione is important in the scavenging of dangerous free radicals during the conversion of carbohydrates to energy in the liver. Taurine is another amino acid produced in the SAM-e metabolism that is important for liver detoxification.

Healthy connective tissue is supported by SAM-e metabolites. Transsulfuration is critical for glucosamine and chondroitin sulfate to work for healthy joints.

There is a reduction of inflammation in the joints with the production of methylthioadenosine that is increased by SAM-e. L-cysteine is also produced by SAM-e; which is an amino acid used to construct a family of sulfur containing compounds (i.e. glutathione) that are used for cartilage, ligaments, tendons, and the matrix for bone production.

The methylation effects of SAM-e are indirectly supportive of brain function. Compounds such as L-dopa, dopamine, epinephrine, and phosphatidylcholine are called neurotransmitters. The donation of methyl groups from SAM-e to make these products is one aspect of what makes the brain function properly.

The methylation from SAM-e facilitates an important conversion in muscles for energy-the recycling of ADP to ATP, and the production of creatine within the muscle. Creatine maximizes the ability of muscles to perform, reduces exercise fatigue, and improves recovery after exercise.

Some scientists believe that DNA imperfections can lead to changes associated with ageing. SAM-e is associated with methylation of DNA and therefore, potentially prevents those imperfections in the DNA from happening.

S-Adenosyl Methionine (SAM-e) is therefore a product that has shown a number of potential benefits for the human body.

Zinc

According to a new systematic review of the evidence, zinc lozenges may shorten the duration of common cold episodes by up to 40%.

The review, published in The Open Respiratory Medicine Journal, reports strong evidence that zinc has a beneficial effect on the common cold duration, depending on the total dosage of zinc.

"Controlled trials that have examined the effect of zinc lozenges on common cold symptoms have reported divergent results," said Dr. Harri Hemila of the University of Helsinki, Finland, who authored the review.

"This meta-analysis shows that a large part of the divergence can be explained by the variation in the total daily dose of zinc that the person obtained from the lozenges," she added.

Interest in the use of zinc for colds grew following the results of a 1984 trial conducted by Eby (Antimicrobial Agents and Chemotherapy 25(1)).

Eby's results suggested that if treatment—consisting of one 23 mg zinc lozenge dissolved in the mouth every second waking hour - commence within 3 days of the development of symptoms of a cold, the average duration of symptoms was reduced by about 7 days.

Hemila carried out a meta-analysis of all the placebo-controlled trials that have examined the effect of zinc lozenges on natural common cold infections.

Of the 13 trials identified, she noted that those using a total daily zinc dose of less than 75 mg found no effect of zinc on the common cold. Hemila reported that trials using zinc daily doses of over 75 mg showed benefit reducing cold duration by 42% on average.

Dr. Hemila concluded "since a large proportion of trial participants have remained without adverse effects, zinc lozenges might be useful for them as a treatment option for the common cold."

CHAPTER 14

A LOOK AT DIETS

The SAD Diet

Most medical professionals refer to SAD as Seasonal Affective Disorder. This is a condition where people do feel sad or depressed due to the lack of stimulation of sunshine.

It is a real disorder often noted in northern latitudes, especially in winter months where there are often days on end when the sun does not shine. This is also why it is called Winter Blues.

Purchasing a ticket to the sunny south – Mexico or Florida – easily cures this disorder. For those who cannot be sunbirds, use of artificial light in the form of a headlamp or light box is just as effective. If patients are resilient to that and want chemical cures, oral antidepressants are another way of treating the disorder.

On the lighter but serious side, another condition that is also called SAD is the Standard American Diet. It is SUPERSIZED in quantity, loaded with processed carbohydrates, loaded with fat and preservatives, and usually contains more protein than is necessary for 5 people for 2 weeks!

America spends more money than any other nation on health. Still, America ranks the lowest in all major industrial nations in terms of life expectancy. According to the most recent World Health Organization report, the United States ranks 24th out of 191 nations, with a life expectancy of 70.0 years, while Japan ranks number 1 with a life expectancy of 74.5 years. If you don't want to be a statistic, you've come to the right place.

Simple Strategies to Healthier Eating

1. Move it and Lose It

The New American diet puts weight control and daily exercise at the broad base of its pyramid, neither of which is mentioned in the traditional USDA model.

A study, which appeared in the April 9, 2003 issue of *The Journal of the American Medical Association*, shows why daily exercise is so beneficial. In it, Harvard researchers report that women who avoid sedentary behaviors, such as watching television more than ten hours per week; and incorporate a thirty-minute brisk walk into their day, reduce the risk of type-2 diabetes by 43% and obesity by 30% compared with women with sedentary lifestyles.

"Aim for 30 minutes a day of moderate physical activity on most days of the week, and lose just 10% of your body weight if you are overweight," says Kathy Berkowitz, RN, past president of the American Association of Diabetes Educators.

"These are not overwhelming changes and can make a huge difference in your health and well-being," she says. Moderate physical activity can include taking the stairs instead of the elevator, or parking a block further from the food store, she says, "and it can be accrued throughout the day in spurts."

2. Take Out Some Insurance in a Pill

Every morning, take a multivitamin, for extra insurance that you are getting all the nutrients your body needs for the day. The new pyramid also encourages us to eat one or two servings of low-fat dairy products a day.

If you don't get your calcium through your diet, you should take a calcium supplement of 500 mg and 500 mg of vitamin D3 to ensure your bones remain strong. This daily recommendation changes often, so you should check with your doctor to ensure that you are receiving the latest recommended for daily intake of calcium and vitamin D.

3. Substitute Whole Grains for Refined Grains

When the waiter asks if you want white or brown rice, say "brown." When he asks what type of bread you want your sandwich on say "wheat" or "rye" --

not white. Better yet, ask for whole grain bread that has not been refined significantly.

Here's why: No matter how you slice it, all breads are not created equal. "There has never been any evidence that large amounts of starches are good for us, but the base of traditional USDA pyramid comprises Wonder Bread, white rice, and pasta," says Willett.

"And now there is good evidence that high amounts of starch can make insulin resistance worse". Insulin resistance means that the body is losing its ability to control blood sugar levels and is a sign that it is not far away.

In the new pyramid, people are encouraged to eat whole-grain foods such as brown rice, whole-grain cereal, and whole wheat or rye bread at most meals. The pyramid puts refined starches such as white rice, white bread, potatoes, and pasta at the top, right next to white sugar.

Whole-grain ingredients to look for when choosing foods include:

- ☑ Whole wheat
- ☑ Whole barley
- ☑ Whole oats
- ☑ Cracked wheat
- ☑ Graham flour
- ☑ Amrinth flour
- ☑ Spelt flour

4. Color-Code Your Plate

The traditional USDA pyramid encourages eating more fruits and vegetables, which is good, but potatoes are not a vegetable, Willett stresses. "They are a major source of starch."

Use a simple color wheel as your guide to the new American Diet. Avoid white foods. Choose a variety of colorful fruits and vegetables. For example, dark leafy green vegetables like spinach and kale are rich in the vitamin folate, which may help prevent colon cancer and heart disease.

Bright red tomatoes are rich in lycopene. Studies have found that men who ate the most tomato-based foods (cooked tomatoes, tomato sauce, and pizza with red sauce) had a 35% lower risk of developing prostate cancer than those who ate the least amount of these foods. Unfortunately, if you have arthritis, tomatoes can make it worse.

When you are loading up your plate, choose dark-green, leafy vegetables, yellow, orange, and red fruits, and vegetables; cooked tomatoes; and citrus fruits.

Willett suggests that you consume veggies in abundance each day and eat two to four servings of fruit a day.

5. Avoid Red Meat

The current dietary pyramid lumps together red meat, fish, nuts, poultry, and legumes. According to Willett, this is not a good call, "There needs to be a distinction between unhealthy and healthy sources of protein in a way that is clear to people."

In Willet's new pyramid, nuts and legumes can be consumed one to three times a day, while fish and chicken can be eaten two or fewer times each week. If you want to eat red meat, it should be consumed sparingly, just once or twice a month. Some would argue that complete elimination of animal protein is even healthier.

6. Choose the Good Fats

"Fat is not a four-letter word," Willett says. "It's true that saturated fats from butter, cheese, milk, and meats are unhealthy, but there are real benefits from unsaturated plant oils."

Monounsaturated and polyunsaturated fats help to lower "bad" cholesterol levels and are found in nuts, avocados, fish, olives, and most plant oils. Healthy fats include olive oil and other plant oils such as soy, canola, corn, safflower, and sunflower oils.

For the new American diet, Willet suggests that these healthy fats should be consumed at most meals. To get started, use olive or canola oil, instead of butter or margarine, but NEVER fry anything, no matter what type of oil you are using. Heating even the good oils to the temperature needed to fry, sauté, etc, changes the character of the oil. This can then cause damage to the body.

Important fats to avoid are the "trans fats," says Dana Greene, MS, a Boston-based nutritionist whose work with overweight children puts her on the front lines of the obesity crisis in the U.S. Fortunately, this fact has now been well publicized and has caught on as a marketing byword.

Trans fatty acids are created when oil, such as corn oil, is hydrogenated so it becomes a solid fat. These hydrogenated fats don't spoil quickly, so they're widely used in cookies, crackers, chips, and other baked goods that you buy in the supermarket.

They're also found in many kinds of margarine and in most fried and fast food. "Trans fat increases levels of 'bad' cholesterol in the bloodstream and decreases levels of 'good' cholesterol," says Greene.

Remember, you don't have to radically change your diet overnight. The best approach is to begin making simple substitutions now, says Melanie Polk, RD, director of nutrition education at the American Institute for Cancer Research in Washington, D.C.

"Making a change in the fat that you use, eating more whole grains, and emphasizing plant-based foods such as beans, nuts, and vegetables are all changes that can be easily made," she says.

Even better, their health benefits are supported by research from around the world!

Diets and Diabetes

There is an epidemic of type-2 diabetes. What can you do to avoid becoming part of this statistic?

Type-2 diabetes, the most common type, occurs when the body uses insulin inefficiently, and can no longer keep blood sugar levels normal. Over the years, this can lead to damage to nerves and blood vessels with heart disease, stroke, blindness, kidney disease, and leg amputation. Type-2 diabetes is preventable.

In people who are overweight, and have higher than normal blood sugar levels - by dropping their weight by just 5% to 7% can delay and possibly prevent type-2 diabetes. Lowering your fat intake, lowering the total caloric intake and doing some kind of exercise such as walking 30 minutes a day on the treadmill, can reduce the risk of type-2 diabetes by 58%. There are several factors that increase the risk of type-2 diabetes – some that you can control and some that you can't.

Type 2 Diabetes Factors You Can't Control:

- ☑ Being over the age of 45
- ☑ Having a close family member with diabetes
- ☑ Being of African-American, American Indian, Asian-American, Pacific Islander, or Hispanic-American/Latino descent
- ☑ Having had diabetes that developed during pregnancy (called gestational diabetes)
- ☑ Having polycystic ovary syndrome –– a condition in women

Factors You Can Control to Prevent Type-2 Diabetes:

- ✓ Being overweight
- ✓ Having blood pressure of 140/90 or higher
- ✓ Having abnormal cholesterol levels –– either HDL "good" cholesterol of less than 35 or triglyceride levels over 250
- ✓ Exercising fewer than three times a week

We all know it is hard to regularly exercise and diet but making the effort is half the battle. Decide what you are going to do and stick to it. Plan what you need to get to do it (exercise pants, t-shirt), find a buddy to exercise with, and decide how you will reward yourself when you have attained your goal weight, and blood level goals.

Being overweight can keep your body from using insulin properly. Insulin is the hormone that allows your body to use sugar for energy. Being overweight can also cause high blood pressure.

Even losing a few pounds can help reduce your risk of developing type-2 diabetes, because it helps your body use insulin more effectively. For example, if you weigh 190 pounds, losing only 10 pounds could make a big difference.

If You Are Overweight or Obese, Choose Sensible Ways to Get in Shape:

✓ Avoid crash diets. Limit the amount of fat you eat.

✓ Increase your physical activity. Aim for at least 30 minutes of exercise most days of the week. This will help your body use insulin more effectively, helping you lower high blood sugars and improving your heart health.

✓ Set a reasonable weight-loss goal, such as losing one pound a week. Aim for a long-term goal of losing 5% to 7% of your total body weight.

What you eat has a big impact on your health. By making wise food choices, you can help control your body weight, blood pressure, and cholesterol. Make those choices most of the time.

✓ Look at the serving sizes of the foods you eat. Reduce serving sizes of main courses such as protein, desserts, and foods high in fat. Increase the amount of fruits and vegetables.

✓ Limit your fat intake to about 25% of your total calories. For example, if your food choices add up to about 2,000 calories a day, try to eat no more than 56 grams of fat. You can check food labels for saturated fat content, too, which increases LDL "bad" cholesterol.

✓ Reduce the number of calories you have each day.

✓ Keep a food and exercise log. Write down what you eat (everything that passes your lips should go in the food diary), how much you exercise - your doctor can review this with you.

✓ Regular exercise tackles several risk factors at once. It helps you lose weight, keeps your cholesterol and blood pressure under control, and helps your body use insulin. Even brisk walking works. Choose activities you enjoy.

A Case Against Very Low Calorie Diets

Diets like the Atkins Diet are very low calorie and very high protein. They are unsuccessful for long-term weight loss and in Dr Atkins case, fatal. If you are one of the people where every diet you try turns into a disaster where at first you lose some pounds and then nothing even when you follow it religiously, you may be feeling like a failure. The truth is -- it's not you. Yo-yo diets don't work, whereas changing ones diet can work.

When you diet, your body realizes your calorie intake has been reduced so the starvation response kicks in and that's the end of your diet. So what is the body's starvation response? Our bodies are like fine-tuned machines, and thus they have a built in safety mechanism, to ensure we don't starve to death.

When we reduce our caloric intake below what is needed these mechanisms kick in, which then reduces the energy we use, ensuring you can survive for a long time with a lower calorie intake. So you cannot win using a diet plan alone.

7 reasons to Avoid Extremely Low Calorie Diets

1. Metabolism

The very first thing the starvation response does is to reduce your metabolic rate. So the lower your intake of calories is the lower your metabolic rate. You can very quickly see that this is going to be a problem since the old formula that you must burn more than you take in cannot occur.

The trouble is the slower your metabolism the harder it is to lose weight. Yet the lower your caloric intake the slower your metabolism will become. Around and around you go, with no hope of winning your battle against the bulge. Your metabolism will reduce itself by at least 20% and can reduce itself up to 45%.

2. Muscle Loss

If you manage to reduce your calories below what your body's metabolism can reduce, then you have another problem, because the very first thing your body is going to burn up is muscle, not fat.

The body's system sees the reduction of your muscle mass as a way to reduce the energy your body needs. After all, muscles require energy to operate. This process is called gluconeogenesis, which means the conversion of muscle into glucose. Your body will even start to devour your heart and internal organs long before it begins to devour your fat cells, which is what you want to get rid of.

Studies have shown that many of those who lose weight using a diet actually lose between 40 to 50% of their lean muscle mass. Diets low in carbohydrates cause the body to dehydrate itself, so between muscle loss and water loss, 80% of your weight loss is from the wrong sources, leaving only 20% of your loss directly related to fat.

3. Decreased Fat Burning Enzyme Activity

When you drop your calories too low, your body's chemistry makeup changes to compensate for the lower calorie intake. It begins to reduce the fat burning enzymes. This allows your body to better store fat in the future.

4. Your Thyroid

The thyroid regulates your metabolism or your metabolic rate. When you severely reduce your calorie intake, the hormone T3 produced by your thyroid is reduced, which results in your body burning fewer calories.

5. Rebound Weight Gain

Anyone who has dieted has experienced rebound weight gain. Initially the pounds fall away, then you hit a plateau where it becomes harder, if not impossible, to lose any weight.

That's because the body's starvation mechanism has come up to full speed. Out of frustration you go off your diet, only to find in no time at all your weight is higher than it was when you began your diet.

That's because now you have a slower metabolism, and your body chemistry has changed to allow for better fat storage so you don't starve again in the future. Now you find yourself weighing more than before you started.

6. Increased Hunger Pains

When you starve your body of calories the cravings or hunger pains kick in trying to get more food into your body. These can become so strong that it becomes impossible to stay on your diet.

7. Decreased Energy

Once your metabolism slows down, so will your energy level. You'll find yourself tired and not able to complete activities that require high energy levels such as your exercise program. You'll also find yourself unable to concentrate on your physical work. Quite frankly, you'll feel lousy!

So the next time you think about trying the latest and greatest high protein very low calorie diet, think about it long and hard because you could end up weighing more than you did to begin with.

A Sensible Diet

For a number of years I worked as a cruise ship physician in between keeping a land based practice going (with 7 other doctors). In that position, I not only saw every type of pathology, but also saw how both crewmembers and passengers dealt with the abundance of excellent food, and it was not always in the most appropriate manner!

I would be presented with diabetics who 'forgot their insulin' and cardiac patients who thought that 'just for this week, I thought it would be ok to eat all the cream sauce and fried food'. As the ship physician, I was not only the doc for the transient passengers, but also the family doc for the crew who were on board for months at a time.

This made me realize that developing a reasonable diet was one way of decreasing my workload, and keeping 'my' crew healthy to enjoy some of the fascinating ports we stopped at. It also gave me lots of material to develop my many novels.

As a crewmember, learning to eat properly on board one of the giant cruise ships is an art. If you are not careful, it is easy to gain weight, and it is hard to lose it. Over the 10 years of working as a ship's doctor, I had my own problems with weight gain.

Whenever I would pass the dessert table, or host a dinner with passengers who wanted "one of each", unfortunately, I often also succumbed to the temptation. In any event, working with many patients shore side, and fellow crewmembers, I developed a fairly simple way of maintaining a healthy weight; whether you are on board a ship, or a land based person wanting to maintain your weight, here is a practical solution.

Since leaving the employ of the cruise lines as a doctor, I have been a guest lecturer on various cruise ships. The caloric intake has not changed, infact I have observed a rather significant increase in gross obesity aboard some of the ships. Four or five desserts and triple helpings have been observed and are necessary to maintain body weights of 400+ pounds! That is the opposite goal of this book. So here goes with various aspects of a sensible diet. I will diverge to mention some other popularized diets along the way.

Dr. Davis's Sensible Diet

No quick weight-loss promises, but stick with this sensible diet, and you will lose weight. Keep it off, and you won't be left with any long-term problems for your liver or heart. Remember the guru of the Atkins diet died from his own diet! Four words you must remember: "Eat right, exercise more."

As I mention in many parts of this book, remember that diet is only one aspect of our lifestyle. Exercise is also very important, as is getting enough sleep and rest between periods of working.

Diet can impact a number of health concerns, from diabetes to allergies; from sinusitis to body odors; from ear infections to irritable bowel syndrome; and even arthritis. One needs to set realistic goals such as losing a maximum of one to two pounds a week. This is the amount that most nutritionists and medically sponsored weight-loss programs counsel as safe, sane, and reasonable.

The trick to successful weight loss is to properly balance the amount of food, and the type of food we eat - the right kinds of carbohydrates, fats, and proteins - which are the building blocks of food. You will never permanently lose weight by cutting out one of the essential building blocks.

This is why if you use the South Beach Diet, Weight Watchers, Jenny Craig, Pritikin Diet, Eat More Diet, Nutri System, African Mango Diet, Zone Diet, or Atkins Diet, you may initially lose weight, but then you gain it all back when you go off the diet.

If you were to stay on the high protein, or zoned carbohydrate diet, then your liver will most likely fail, your kidneys would stop filtering, and there is even new evidence that some aspects of Alzheimer's disease may start from these extreme diets, and the bouncing weight loss/gain.

This diet can work on a ship or nowhere near a ship. It is a bit like mixing foods from Spain, France, Italy, India, Greece, and parts of the Middle East. Let's have a more detailed look.

Protein

In this diet, protein should be limited to 20% of your diet, and vegetable proteins from foods like beans and soybeans should be substituted for animal protein as often as possible.

A vegetarian buffet at lunch or a vegetable curry is a good option! Mushrooms are a high source of protein and very low in calories. Sunflower seeds and other nuts are good protein, but they do have high fat content, even though it's good fat. If you must eat animal protein, choose baked or boiled fish, boiled chicken or low fat dairy. These are ALL scientifically based suggestions. Make sure you eliminate red meat (beef, veal, pork, etc).

Fats

This diet allows 30% of your calorie intake from fats, as long as most of that amount is from monounsaturated oils such as olive oil and foods high in what are known as omega-3 fatty acids: oily fishes like salmon, sardines, or mackerel, flax seeds, and walnuts. The fats we have to avoid are the ones in fried foods that change good fats to bad fats - in other words, nothing fried.

Carbohydrates

For this Sensible Diet, complex carbohydrates should account for up to 50% of your calorie intake, and as much of these as possible from unrefined grains and vegetables (higher in complex carbohydrates). These release glucose (sugar) into the bloodstream more slowly, and therefore, won't as readily cause rapid spikes after meals that make you want to eat more, and send fat into storage in your liver.

Good carbs include apples, baked beans, oatmeal, and stone-ground whole-grains, whole grain pasta, brown rice, etc. Interestingly, while white rice is banned, red, brown basmati, and plain brown rice are acceptable, because they release glucose at a reasonable rate when eaten with other foods (that does not include pouring butter over the rice!). As a result, you will not gain weight.

Fiber

As mentioned elsewhere in the book, I again recommend that you eat at least 40 grams of fiber a day, which isn't hard to achieve if you eat fruits (not fruit juice), vegetables (all kinds), and whole grains (Quinoa, Millet, Spelt, Rye, Wheat, Oat, etc.)

Avoid milk and consume limited amounts of cheese and other dairy products. First, they are usually high in fat, unless you drink skim milk. Secondly, a great many of the world's population -- particularly those of Asian and African-descent -- have some degree of difficulty digesting these because they are usually lactose intolerant and others may be allergic to milk protein.

These intolerances can lead to a host of problems for the body. Furthermore, you may be surprised to learn you don't need milk after you have been weaned from the breast. After all how many adult cows do you see suckling other cows protein a day.

Calcium

Even without dairy products, we can keep up with our calcium needs with this diet. Ingesting too much protein leeches calcium out of the body, so if you consume less protein, then you need less calcium.

All you need is ONE protein meal a day. Non-dairy sources include sardine bones, which are usually canned without removing the bones, leafy greens, broccoli, and various sea vegetables such as nori, dulse, and kombu (remember the sushi bar when going out for a meal). In addition, tofu, sesame seeds, calcium-fortified orange juice, and fortified soymilk, can be good calcium sources.

The Science Behind Why This Diet Works

Complex carbohydrates, beans, vegetables, and grains are converted to glucose and mainly used for energy. The brain likes its energy from carbohydrates. However, too many carbs do not make us brainy -- they make us overweight.

Not enough carbohydrates send us into ketosis, in which the body retrieves energy from fat stores and muscles. However, ketosis is detrimental to our health over the long term, principally because of toxins produced, a rise in lipids, cholesterol levels, and calcium depletion. The best carbohydrates are beans, unrefined grains, and vegetables - these are the foods that release glucose slowly. Medically speaking, these carbohydrates are said to have a low glycemic index.

Fats and oils are more concentrated sources of energy than carbohydrates, but they need to be chemically converted into glucose, so the body can use them. Although fat has a bad name in today's collective health consciousness, some fat is essential. The key is that we need the right balance. Too much fat makes us fat, as well as sets us up for a number of diseases such as diabetes, heart disease and cancer.

However, not enough fat, and we may run into problems too, such as skin diseases, hair loss, and susceptibility to infection. Remember this does NOT mean you should eat French fries—it does, however, mean more olive oil on your salad.

We need proteins to build, maintain, and repair the body. But they can be converted to glucose, and therefore, serve as an energy source when needed. They are composed of 20 amino acids – 10 of which must be supplied by foods on a regular basis.

Ingesting too much protein increases the workload of the digestive system, and strains the liver, and kidneys. Too little will cause malnutrition, increased susceptibility to infection, and possibly early death, so a proper balance is what one needs.

Exercise

Exercise is a key component of this program. You don't have to be a gym rat, but you do need regular exercise. It consumes calories and in time can change the basic weight-loss equation in your favor helping you to keep off the pounds over the long term. It triggers the metabolic rate to notch up, and regularly get rid of the extra pounds, even when you are not exercising.

Doing work around a ship, factory, in your garden, or even heavy manual work is not the kind of exercise we need to add to our regime to lose and keep the weight off. The same applies to everyone.

No matter what type of work you do heavy lifting or not, you need at least 20-30 minutes of continuous aerobic exercise, a minimum of 3 times a week, to keep the heart healthy and keep the weight off. Many suggest up to 6 times a week fast walking, elliptical, treadmill, stair stepper, swimming (excellent), yoga, etc. are all ways of doing that.

There is a vast amount of scientific evidence that shows that a mostly vegetarian diet with small amounts of animal products are the healthiest diets for lowering mortality from heart disease and cancer, and indeed, all causes. This is a diet for the long term—not just to get a few pounds off in the spring for that swimsuit in the summer.

I place a lot of emphasis on your responsibility for your own health, because you can't have someone standing over you all the time telling you what to eat, and what to do. A personal trainer or buddy can help keep you exercising, and friends can remind you of what you are eating, but ultimately, it is you that has to pick up the fork or the weight machine.

Oh and yes, by the way, since you are reading this book I can only assume that your health is important to you, and that you are looking to stay healthy or become healthier. So take these suggestions as just that, suggestions - the rest is up to you - and good luck.

The American Diet

It's as if famed Harvard nutritionist Walter Willet, M.D., Dr.PH, MPH, took a trip around the world. But instead of collecting postcards or campy souvenirs, he amassed healthy eating styles and strategies from across the globe.

From Greece and southern Italy, he borrowed the liberal use of olive oil and a glass of wine with dinner. From China and Japan, he picked up a reliance on plant-based proteins, such as soy. From the Latin American countries, he adapted their generous use of whole-grain foods and more active lifestyle.

Instead of putting his souvenirs in a traditional scrapbook, Willet used them to build a new eating pyramid -- the new American Diet, which he published, in the book *Eat, Drink and Be Healthy: The Harvard Medical School Guide to Healthy Eating.*

The Eating Melting Pot

America is once again a melting pot -- this time of eating wisdom and traditions from around the world. Moreover, it's about time. Certain nutrition experts consider the traditional United States Department of Agriculture (USDA) Food Guide Pyramid as outdated. Others go as far as saying that it may be contributing to the soaring rates of obesity in this country.

Here's why: The current USDA guidelines encourage large amounts of carbohydrates in the American Diet. They don't distinguish between types of fat and they lump red meat, chicken, nuts and legumes together. Most new research shows that a plant-based diet is advantageous for its level of fat, and the complex carbohydrates that it portends.

By contrast, the newly revamped eating pyramid created by Willett emphasizes

- ☑ White meat over red
- ☑ Whole grains over refined
- ☑ Plant oils over spreads made with saturated fat

He says his pyramid, which is based on 20-years of research, could someday lower our rates of heart disease and diabetes – if enough Americans post it on their refrigerator door.

How? Here's just one example: Certain carbohydrates carry a high glycemic load, which means they increase blood sugar levels in the body too rapidly. Whole grain foods lead to a slower and lower peak of blood sugar.

Traditional American diets are filled with high-glycemic-index foods, which cause quick and strong increases in blood sugar levels, and they have been linked to an increased risk for both diabetes, and heart disease. "That's why it's healthier to separate whole grains from other carbohydrates," Willett says.

Indeed, early evidence shows that people, who follow the new American diet or similar diets with many of the precepts of the new American diet, do significantly improve their health. Researchers at the Harvard School of Public Health found that men who followed the new American diet lowered their overall risk of a major chronic disease by 20%. The same study found women lowered their overall risk of a major chronic disease by 11%.

So how do you start if you're interested in following the new American diet? Good news – You don't have to jet off to the Mediterranean or Hong Kong to learn this new style of eating. Just follow the simple strategies we've provided. Use them at home and out at restaurants.

Biblical Diet - The Maker's Diet

Next time you are craving a snack or unsure what to prepare for dinner, ask yourself, what would Jesus eat? Still unsure? A new diet called the Maker's Diet promises to clear it up for you.

This 40-day guide is built on principles first described in the Bible. But some nutritionists aren't so sure that anyone can say for certain exactly what Jesus ate and whether or not it was good for him.

The Maker's Diet: the 40-Day Health Experience That Will Change Your Life Forever encompasses physical, spiritual, mental, and emotional health. Written by Jordan S. Rubin, NMD, PhD, this new eating plan is rich in whole, organic foods and eventually includes red meat, carbs, and some saturated fats.

The catch is that all of these foods must be consumed in their natural state -- unprocessed, unrefined, and untreated with pesticides or hormones. Carb is not a four-letter word in the Maker's Diet -- starches and sugars are allowed as long as they are consumed in their natural, unrefined form such as brown rice, fermented whole grain sourdough bread, oats, and barley.

The diet is complete with low carbohydrate, high-fiber foods such as broccoli, cauliflower, berries, grapes, certain seeds, nuts, grains, and legumes. The diet permits natural fats, including those found in fish, cod liver oil, and the saturated fat found naturally in butters, cheeses, milk, and creams. The Maker's Diet includes weekly partial fast days in each phase of the diet.

More Than Food

Reducing toxins is a key component of the Maker's Diet and that includes avoiding water, toothpaste treated with fluoride, cavities filled with mercury, and overexposure to electromagnetic fields such as excess X-rays, cell phones, and living near power lines or microwave use. Rubin also recommends beginning and ending each day with a prayer for healing or thanks. Hygiene in the form of hand washing before meals, after using the bathroom and at other crucial times is also part of the new plan.

"While most people lose an average of 10 to 15 pounds in the first 40 days, The Maker's Diet goes far beyond a weight loss program, providing people with a lifelong roadmap for achieving and maintaining total wellness," Rubin says.

Maker's Diet in Action

The Maker's Diet is broken down into three, 2-week stages. The first stage is the most restrictive, prohibiting many commercial dairy products, chlorinated tap water, many fats and oils, and all carbs. As the weeks progress, more foods are introduced, including red meat, carbs and saturated fats.

Nutritionists Sound Off

"I don't know of any data that suggests that organic is better than other produce, but it's more expensive," says Ruth Kava, PhD, RD, and Director of Nutrition at the American Council on Science and Health in New York.

" 'Organic' and 'natural' have that 'good-for-you buzz,' but there are a lot of natural poisons and carcinogens, so that part of this marketing ploy does not get me too excited." The Maker's Diet strongly encourages consuming organic fruits, and vegetables.

She adds that in the distant past people were unaware of vitamins. "We have come a long way in terms of our knowledge, and I don't think that should be ignored," she says.

"One of the things [Rubin] said is that our ancestors enjoyed exceptional health, but I don't know how he knows that from the Bible," she says. It is also well known that people in the era of the Bible died at much younger ages, usually from infectious diseases.

Once one had a disease in biblical times, either you had an incredibly strong immune system to fight it off, or with a combo of natural foods and local herbs the patient could fight it off. Otherwise, you just died of the malady.

Still, Kava says certain things in the Maker's Diet are reasonable -- healthful even. "It's a mixed bag," she says. "He picked up on a lot of the faddy, crazy things about modern lifestyles such as danger from electromagnetic fields and avoiding fluoride in the water supply, but hand washing is important and reasonable."

Victoria Shanta-Retelny, RD, a dietitian at Northwestern Memorial Hospital's Wellness Institute in Chicago, is less approving about the new, old diet. "The basic premise of The Maker's Diet, which is a '40-day health experience that will change your life forever,' begs skepticism," she said.

"The plan is gimmicky as it focuses on fasting one day per week, which I don't recommend as a general guideline because we are not sure what a person's specific health concerns are, such as diabetes," she says. This could be extremely dangerous to a diabetic patient.

What's more, there are a myriad of supplements that the diet touts as essential, she says. "One of them, extra-virgin coconut oil, is marketed as the 'healthier oil' when the nutrition literature does not support this," she says. If anything, she says, "coconut oil is 92% saturated fat – the type that can clog arteries." Coconut oil is known to be good for applying to skin, but never advised for oral consumption by humans.

Shanta-Retelny says the supplements and cleansing agents are not necessary if you are eating a healthy diet, and not eliminating food groups that are high in fiber, vitamins, and minerals.

So is there any population that may benefit from the Maker's Diet?

"Since this diet is based (in part) on kosher practices, it may be better for a strict Orthodox Jewish population, who may practice holistic living, but I would not recommend it to the general population," she says.

Bland Diet

Chickens and many other animals eat very small amounts on a regular basis. Thus the expression – "a chicken picking at its food." It is not always necessary to eat very small amounts of food regularly, but it is important to eat several times a day but in smaller quantities.

THINGS TO EAT

- ✓ Baked or boiled Potatoes
- ✓ Boiled eggs (only the whites)
- ✓ Creamed soups-creamed with tofu
- ✓ Non-citrus fruit (No OJ)
- ✓ Very Grainy Bread
- ✓ Fish & Chicken - - baked or grilled, not fried
- ✓ Multi grain cereal, cold or cooked
- ✓ Salads (with no dressing)
- ✓ Only Lukewarm or Cool Things
- ✓ Water, Apple Juice, Milk-like drinks

THINGS NOT TO EAT:

- ✓ Fried Things
- ✓ Red Meat
- ✓ Spicy Things
- ✓ Very Hot Things
- ✓ Very Cold Things
- ✓ Coffee, Sodas
- ✓ Anything Else You Notice Bothers Your Stomach

Japanese Diet

The waiter gently places a lacquered mahogany box before you. A delicate piece of grilled salmon rests in one quadrant. A tangle of seaweed glistens in the center. Crimson tuna sashimi accented with a thimble of potent wasabi shines in a neighboring corner; a half moon of white rice completes this manicured mosaic.

Although most modern Japanese people don't eat this way on a daily basis, this is typical of a meal eaten in a traditional restaurant. It's a feast not only for the palate but also for the eyes: a portrait of order, clarity, and simplicity.

"The Japanese have an aesthetic appetite. Enormous pleasure is taken in the presentation of food," says Elizabeth Andoh, owner of A Taste of Culture, a Tokyo school that educates non-Japanese businesspeople in the food and customs of Japan.

The Japanese pay as much attention to the menu selections, which often feature sea foods in season, as they do to the serving plates that are used, whether lacquer, ceramic, or bamboo.

Indeed, at formal Japanese meals, presentation is key. For added appeal, "you might see garnishes of leaves and flowers from the garden," says Lucy Seligman, who teaches Japanese cooking in Richmond, California to those of us living in North America, nations of dashboard diners, and connoisseurs of cubicle cuisine, such mealtime mindfulness may seem downright foreign, not to mention time-consuming.

But American eaters would do well to turn off their TVs and cell phones, and follow the Japanese lead by spending more time enjoying meals, especially if they're watching their weight.

Why All the Fuss?

During the sixth century, the religion of the land was declared as Buddhism. It was at this time that eating the flesh of fowl and "four-legged" was forbidden.

The Japanese meal is prepared "to be eaten with the eyes." In an effort to make this meatless cuisine more appealing and satisfying, they started to focus on elegance.

Today many Japanese eat meat. However, they still focus on making sure their food is beautifully displayed, in the same manner you would expect it to be presented in a fine restaurant.

Besides the visual appeal of traditional Japanese meals, there is also an element of deep respect. According to ancient Buddhist principles, "eating should be a spiritual experience that gives you a moment of calm during the day," says Donald Altman, a former Buddhist monk and author of *Art of the Inner Meal: Eating as a Spiritual Path*.

According to the Japanese principle of eating with the eyes, you'll get more satisfaction per calorie by paying attention to presentation. For example, a small serving of tofu will be less apt to leave you hungering for more when sliced, well flavored and fanned on a pretty plate. A half-cup of frozen yogurt, really satisfies when it is served in a beautiful bowl, and topped with a strawberry.

Even if you don't have time to artfully arrange your meals, "at least put your food on a plate rather than eating it out of the take-out carton," says Daniel Stettner, PhD, director of psychology in the department of preventive and nutritional medicine at William Beaumont Hospital in Birmingham, Mich.

According to Japanese tradition, a meal should be a meaningful sensory experience, he says. "It's not about how fast you can get it down so you can go on to the next thing."

"Feeding your senses and thinking of mealtimes as stress breaks can help make your meal more satisfying and slow you down enough to consume fewer calories," says Stettner. "Satiety is often absent when people wolf down their food, or when they are very distracted."

It takes 20 minutes for your brain to respond to increased glucose levels and get the "I'm full" message, he says. "If you were to eat a reasonable amount of food in less than 20 minutes, you could still be hungry." In other words, if you took more than 20 minutes to eat the same amount of food, you'd likely feel fuller. "

Eating on the run is also an efficient way to consume loads of fat, and calories without even realizing it. For example, consider a McDonald's ham, egg, and cheese breakfast bagel. According to nutritional information furnished by the company, in just a few hasty bites during your morning commute you'll consume roughly 40% of the calories and sodium found in the average 2000-calorie diet, and 27% of the allotted saturated fat.

American-style speed eating can also leave you empty emotionally. "What you're lacking in fulfillment, you may make up by indiscriminately nibbling at different times of the day," says Stettner.

Calories on the Rise

With habits like these, it's no wonder the U.S. Department of Agriculture's statistics show that the average daily caloric intake of Americans has risen from 1,854 calories to 2,002 calories during the last 20 years.

That significant increase -- 148 calories per day -- works out to an extra 15 pounds a year. And now, with the epidemic of obesity, triple those calories to see what the average American is consuming.

Meanwhile, according to the American Institute for Cancer Research in Washington, D.C., from 1975 to 1993, the caloric intake in Japan declined an average of 192 calories per day.

The typical Japanese diet has remained comparatively low in fat, weighing in at roughly 9% less than the typical American one. In addition, according to the World Health Organization, the life expectancy in Japan is 74.5 years, which is 4-1/2 years longer than that of Americans.

Mealtime and Mindfulness

The Japanese tradition of mealtime mindfulness probably contributes to this stellar statistic. So how can you translate these Japanese practices to your own life? Here, are three thoughts:

1. Take 20

Set a specific time for eating. Say at least 20 minutes each -- for meals. "Think, as I'm going through my day, I need to schedule time for me as much as I'm scheduling time for others," says Stettner. Go ahead and jot lunch into your calendar if you must.

Your mission: To truly experience the food you eat. Consider those 20-minute time-outs as personal self-care breaks that can help you avoid overeating.

2. Eliminate Distractions

To get even more fulfillment from meals, eliminate distractions like the television and the phone. After all, that's what answering machines are for. "Light a candle, make it special," says Altman. "Do something that helps you appreciate the moment."

3. Use Food to Nourish Your Body

Sit down and let the meal nourish your mind, body, and spirit. According to Japanese tradition, less can be so much more if you don't let your meals consume you.

Importing "The Japanese Way" American-Style

1. A Rice Base

The Japanese diet includes large quantities of rice. In fact, it's six times more per person than the average American diet. Serve a small bowl of rice with most meals. It will fill you up and has few calories. Unfortunately, the Japanese and many other Asian cultures use white rice, which are empty carb calories. So, instead of the white rice, use brown rice that has all the nutrients of rice plus the fiber that eats up the carb calories for you.

2. Veggie Pleasure

The Japanese diet is a vegetable based diet to a great extent. Mixed vegetables simmer and are included in almost every meal. These include green beans, red bell peppers, zucchini, burdock, onions, tomatoes, lettuce, green peppers, eggplant, bamboo, carrots, spinach, beets, shoots, turnips, shiitake mushrooms, bok choy, a great variety of seaweeds and sweet potatoes.

A single meal can include four or more varieties, which are healthy choices. Unlike the Japanese, eat these healthy vegetables raw or lightly steamed, rather than simmering the veggies in a seasoned broth (too much salt).

3. Add a Little Fish

Include omega-3, rich fatty fish, such as fresh tuna, salmon, sardines, herring, or mackerel to your diet. These are all a good source of omega-3 fatty acids, which have plenty of the healthy fats. So next time, avoid the red meat that contains saturated fats, which clog the arteries and replace with a little fish for some overall heart health.

4. Soy is Good

The Japanese diet includes soy in a great variety of presentations. Snack foods such as edamame beans and dried tofu jerky are an easy way to include some of the healthy soybeans in your diet. There are of course bits of tofu put into classical miso soup (the little white cubes) and in other Japanese soups. Tofu is a good alternative to red meat, containing a higher percent of protein than animal protein, without all the fat.

There are a multitude of types of tofu and it can be added to or made the main ingredient of a meal. Visit your local Asian grocery store and head toward the refrigerated section where a whole host of soy based products can be found and are usually much less costly than those in a general western-based supermarket. Try to avoid the ubiquitous candy section in those stores or the pastries, which will nullify all the good found in the soy-based products.

5. Delicious Desserts

A traditional Japanese dessert is made up of seasonal fruits that are sliced or peeled and arranged in an appealing presentation on a plate. The occasional soy custard is okay, but you must make sure the portions are small, and no more than once a week.

6. Seek Out Healthy Choices

As mentioned above, swap white rice for brown rice, an ancient Japanese power food that's high in fiber. It is healthy to reduce the sodium in your diet. The traditional Japanese diet is too high in sodium with pickled foods, miso, soy paste, and regular soy sauce.

Don't bring the bad habit of salt into your Americanized Japanese diet. Simply reduce the amount of soy sauce you use, and purchase a low-sodium soy sauce. If you want to live longer and do it in a healthier state, the Japanese diet has some things to offer. You'll also be slimmer for it. Don't be afraid to experiment and mix it up a little with vegetables, fish, brown rice, and other things that you can add to your basic diet.

The Chinese Diet

Scan the menu at your local Chinese restaurant and you're apt to find dozens of meat-centered dishes -- General Tso's chicken, orange beef, twice-fried pork. But don't be fooled. Most Chinese people living in China don't eat such meat-centered diets. This is made for the American Chinese food menu.

For centuries, for religious, economic and historic reasons, the traditional Chinese diet has been primarily vegetarian -- featuring lots of vegetables, rice, and soybeans; and containing only shavings of meat for flavoring. Many Chinese simply can't afford mega slabs of meat -- or the cooking oil with which to prepare it.

Just as Americans might ask, "Where's the beef?" when they visit a traditional Chinese restaurant in China; the traditional Chinese might wonder, "Where are the vegetables when they visit a Chinese restaurant in the U.S.

"Even I forget just how healthy Chinese food really is until my mother visits from Taiwan," says Tan, who came to the U.S. more than a decade ago. "My mother will use one-third pound of meat to feed six people."

Indeed, the traditional Chinese diet is far healthier than the traditional American diet, which often features meat as the focus of the meal, says T. Colin Campbell, PhD, professor of nutritional biochemistry at Cornell University in Ithaca, N.Y.

But you don't have to travel to rural parts of China to eat healthy. Simply incorporate the Chinese way of eating into your diet, which can be done no matter where you are -- whether you're dining at a restaurant or preparing Chinese dishes at home.

The Meat Myth

"Unlike the meat-heavy plates featured in many Chinese restaurants in the U.S., the traditional Chinese diet consists mainly of plant foods, small amounts of fish, poultry, and only occasionally red meat," says Campbell, the director of the Cornell-China-Oxford Project on Nutrition, Health, and Environment.

Campbell has been involved in a long-term study comparing the diets of rural China with average American ones. He has been tracking the eating habits of people living in 100 Chinese rural villages since the early 1980s. According to Campbell's research, the traditional Chinese diet is comprised of only 20% animal foods -- far less than the amount in the typical American diet.

As a result, the Chinese diet contains a formidable team of disease-fighting antioxidants and plant-based nutrients called phytochemicals -- all of which contribute to a healthier way of eating.

Rural China

In rural China, the rates of major chronic diseases including breast, colon, and rectal cancer are mere fractions of those reported in the United States, unless they are located near to one of the toxic chemical plants or the population has acquired a western type diet.

Campbell says, "There are some regions in China in which breast cancer and heart disease are almost unknown. Moreover, type-2 diabetes is also much less prevalent, as is bone-weakening osteoporosis, even though the Chinese consume far fewer dairy products than we do in the U.S."

Just what do the traditional Chinese actually eat? "For breakfast, it's often congee, a thin rice porridge," says Qin, a 31-year-old who grew up in a rural village near Shanghai. "Lunch might be rice with vegetables flavored with bits of pork, even at school." And dinner? "

"My mother always served rice and four other kinds of dishes, which we call main dishes. At least one main dish would be all vegetables -- different kinds of greens, sweet potatoes, or tomatoes. The rest were vegetables or tofu with a little bit of beef or pork for flavor."

Importing "The Chinese Way" American-Style

Crowding your plate with complex carbohydrates, such as brown rice and vegetables, and using meat as more of a flavoring for these healthier options, is the Chinese recipe for good health. The best part is you can work this healthy diet into your everyday meals, no matter where you are. Just follow these five tips.

1. Out for Chinese Food?

Enjoy! But skip the deep-fried Chinese-American fare, such as sweet and sour pork. Instead, head for the vegetarian section of the menu and eat the way the Chinese do.

Look for entrees made with napa cabbage, bok choy, spinach, and broccoli, which are packed with Vitamin A and C, as well as fiber, and phytochemicals.

Even though fresh or lightly steamed is better, Chinese vegetables are usually stir fried, which is a quick-cooking technique that tends to preserve some of the water-soluble vitamins (such as A and C).

If the menu indicates that the vegetables will be steamed, order them lightly steamed to minimize nutrient loss during cooking.

If meat is a must, order your chicken or beef stir fried (not deep fried) with vegetables, snow peas, green and red peppers, string beans, or zucchini. Still hungry? Consider an extra serving of brown rice.

2. Dining Elsewhere? Or at Home?

Give vegetables, and grains (including brown rice or whole grain pasta) entree status. Consider meat a flavoring rather than the main attraction. To safeguard your intentions, buy meat in quarter pound packages or ask the butcher to divvy up a larger package for you or use one of the vegetarian meat substitutes.

As you will recall when I was dining in a Chinese Buddhist monastery near Shanghai, I was assured that all the 'meat' dishes were all vegetarian. The taste was incredibly close to the 'real thing'. My fellow travelers commented on how tender the 'meat' was, and how it did not taste like the fried rat they had been served the night before!

Once a week, it's a good idea to go all out and have a totally vegetarian meal, such as one of the many Chinese vegetarian meat substitutes, vegetable lasagna or baked white or sweet potatoes with vegetarian toppings.

According to the American Institute for Cancer Research (AICR), vegetables, fruits, whole grains, and beans should make up two-thirds or more of the meal, like they have had in rural China for centuries. Animal foods should make up a minimal amount of the diet. Of course, research institutes recommend 100% plant based diets as the most healthful.

But before you pat yourself on the back for eating your broccoli, take heed. Variety is key. "Each fruit, vegetable, or grain has its own profile of cancer-protective substances that tend to work as a team," says Melanie Polk, RD, an AICR spokeswoman.

In short, when it comes to disease-proofing your diet, eat more plant foods like the Chinese do. For the best health insurance, expand your repertoire to include vitamin-packed Chinese favorites, such as bok choy, kale, Swiss chard, sweet potatoes, bean sprouts, spinach, and eggplant.

3. Sneak in Fruits and Veggies

This is a good way to heighten the produce quotient of your diet without realizing it. For example, the Chinese stir-fry is a sneaky way to get a host of vegetables all in one sitting.

Try these North American ways to do the same thing:

- ☑ Top off your morning cereal or yogurt with bananas, berries, or peaches.
- ☑ Layer sandwiches with dark leafy greens such as spinach and watercress.
- ☑ Order your chicken or fish sandwich with extra lettuce, tomato, and other veggies.
- ☑ Roll bean sprouts, shredded cabbage, and slices of green or red pepper into tortillas or flat bread; heap salsa onto low-fat tortilla

chips; toss petite peas, tomatoes, onion, celery, carrots, and peppers into a salad.

☑ Tuck mushrooms, peppers, zucchini, onions, and carrots into pasta sauce, 'meat' loaf, soup, stew, and chili.

4. When You Eat Meat American-Style

If you are going to eat meat the American way, make sure your star attraction is low-fat cuts.

Limit portions to 1-ounce - this is about the size of a CD disk. Trim all visible fat from the meat before cooking: You'll save an average of 11 grams of fat (roughly 100 calories) per serving by pre-trimming, which prevents fat from migrating into the meat during cooking. Also, skip the skin, and you'll save an additional 100 calories per 3-ounce serving.

5. Choose Fruit for Dessert

Cloying concoctions such as brownies, chocolate cheesecake, and pecan pie, after a meal, are a bit of a head-scratcher to the Chinese. Their culture doesn't participate in the post-meal ritual we call heavy dessert. Fresh fruit, on the other hand, is the unofficial national treat of China.

Of course, because fruit has no fat and fewer calories than most classic Western desserts, fruit is a much better nutritional deal. It offers up disease-fighting nutrients, such as fiber, folic acid, in addition to vitamins A and C.

As you can see, with a few diet modifications, "the Chinese way" is easily available for importing. All it takes is an adventurous palate, some inventiveness in the kitchen, and the desire to stay healthy for the long haul. "The closer you get to a plant-based diet," says Campbell, "the better off you'll be."

If you want to enjoy the health benefits of the Chinese diet; all you have to do is employ most of the traditional Chinese diet, and you can enjoy longevity, healthier weight, fewer diseases, and less heart disease.

Mediterranean Diet

If you want to know the secrets to a long life, ask Ancel Keys, age 96. Don't be surprised if he points to tonight's meal of roasted potatoes, steamed broccoli, baked cod fillets with lemon juice and olive oil, and a glass of white wine.

It's typical Mediterranean diet, befitting to the man who was first to promote the health benefits of the Mediterranean diet. As a young scientist more than 50 years ago, Ancel Keys showed that heart disease is rare in countries like Southern Italy, Greece, Southern France, the Middle East, and North Africa, where people had free access to fresh fruits, and vegetable, as well as olive oil.

Compare this to places like the United States where plates are filled with cheese, beef, and other foods that are high in saturated fat. Heart disease is the leading cause of death for those who eat like this.

Thanks to Keys' efforts, cooking and eating the Mediterranean diet has become synonymous with good health. However, recently the cuisine that's touted as the healthiest in the world has taken some knocks.

In the past few years, Italian scientists have linked bread, pasta, and rice made from refined grains (think white bread) to an increased risk of certain cancers, particularly thyroid, colon, and stomach cancers.

Two separate nutrition studies published in 1998 found similar results. Meanwhile, the Center for Science in the Public Interest (CSPI) issued a scathing report that they found on the food served in Italian restaurants. Menu staples like fettuccine Alfredo are often laden with as much saturated fat as three pints of butter-almond ice cream. A serving of fried calamari may have the cholesterol equivalent of a four-egg omelet.

When a Good Diet Goes Bad

Those entrées are a long way from the foods that Keys first promoted. The original Mediterranean diet was that eaten by rural villagers on the Greek Island of Crete. The Mediterranean diet was nearly vegetarian, with occasional fish, and was rich in green vegetables and fruits.

People living on Crete got more than one-third of their calories from fat, most of it from olive oil, which is rich in monounsaturated fatty acids. They also consumed wine every day.

Americanized Mediterranean Diet

Unfortunately, something got lost in the translation when these traditional diets were brought to America. "They may call it Italian, but it's very different from the food we studied," says Keys, who for the past three decades has divided his time between Minneapolis and a small village 40 miles south of Naples, Italy, on the shores of the Mediterranean. "What happens here (USA) is that we add a great deal of meat, sugar, and a lot of cream sauces."

Jayne Hurley, RD, the senior nutritionist who helped conduct the survey of Italian restaurants for CSPI, agrees. "We're not saying Italian food is unhealthy," says Hurley. "But the food we saw had been Americanized."

For example, while the traditional diets used cheese and meat sparingly as a condiment, the American versions are typically loaded with them. Nancy Harmon Jenkins, a food writer and author of *The Mediterranean Diet Cookbook* explains, "Spaghetti, as served in the United States, often includes a generous helping of grated cheese and up to a pound of ground meat."

"Traditional food can easily become corrupted from simple ignorance of the cook," says Paula Wolfert, a San Francisco-based author of several Mediterranean-style cookbooks. At one restaurant she visited, Moroccan kabobs were made with pork. "The population of Morocco is predominantly Muslim, and they don't eat pork products," she says. Kabobs are traditionally made from lamb, chicken, or fish.

What's more, many breads and pastas are no longer prepared the traditional way. Refined flours were never part of the original Mediterranean diet, says K. Dun Gifford, president of the Oldways Preservation and Exchange Trust, which is a food education and policy group based in Massachusetts.

The diet that Keys studied, was one eaten by poor farmers and laborers, who ate whole grain breads and pastas. "White flour was more expensive than whole grain flour," says Gifford, who has earned a reputation as a crusader for back-to-the-basics cooking. "We call it peasant bread, or rough country bread."

Recapturing the Mediterranean Ideal

With a few careful choices, you can still treat yourself to one of the world's healthiest and most delicious cuisines. Here are four tips to get you started.

1. Fill Your Plate With Fresh Fruits and Vegetables

The people of Crete were called mangifolia, which means "leaf-eaters," because they consumed so many leafy green vegetables, foraged from the steep hillsides of the island.

Fruits, and vegetables are low in calories and fat, and they are very rich in nutrients, including cancer-fighting antioxidants. Climbing the hillsides for your food also incorporated the exercise needed for the healthy lifestyle.

2. If You're Dining Out, Look for Entrees With Plenty of Vegetables and No Cream

Try vegetarian pasta tossed in olive oil and a little Parmesan cheese, for instance, or grilled fish served with steamed vegetables.

3. When Buying Bread, Choose Loaves Made With Whole Grains and Flours

"Refined foods cause blood sugar levels to spike because they are so easily digested, " says David Jacobs Jr, PhD, professor of epidemiology at the University of Minnesota in Minneapolis. "Less processed, whole grains provide a more sustained level of energy over a longer period, making them more healthful," says Keys.

4. For Dessert, Choose Something That Provides One Serving of Fruit

At his home in Minneapolis, Keys ends his meal with a dessert that perfectly reflects the Mediterranean diet: baked apple slices, sprinkled lightly with cinnamon.

5. Eat Plenty of Nuts, Seeds, Legumes

For protein include healthy nuts, and seeds in your diet, as well as, legumes, some seafood, and yogurt.

6. Eat Foods in Season

According to Eve Adamson, co-author of *Mediterranean Women Stay Slim, Too*, you should eat foods that are in season and grown locally. Avoid foods that are processed. Some Canadians are challenging themselves to the 100–

mile rule, which means you buy only foods that originated within 100 miles of where you live.

7. Control Your Portions

The Mediterranean diet focuses on high quality foods in small portions. When you are eating delicious tasting food, your senses are satisfied, and therefore, you should only need a small portion.

8. Use Olive Oil

In the Mediterranean, olive oil is used on everything from breads to pastas, to fish, to pastries. It's the main fat in the Mediterranean diet, and it's a healthy fat. But remember, they do not fry or otherwise alter the olive oil. Instead, they sprinkle it on food.

Researchers at the Monell Chemical Senses Center in Philadelphia found that oleocanthal, a compound in olive oil, might reduce inflammation, which could help prevent conditions like heart disease, diabetes, arthritis, Alzheimer's, and autoimmune diseases, as well as certain cancers.

9. Incorporate Omega-3 Fatty Acids

Healthy Omega-3 fatty acids are found in abundance in the Mediterranean diet. They are filled with healthy benefits that include reduced incidence of blood clots, strokes, hypertension, and heart attacks, as well as some forms of cancer. In reality, one wants to include Omega-6 and Omega-9, which are often found in many of the same foods.

The Portfolio Diet: Lowers Cholesterol

For lower cholesterol, fit four cholesterol-fighting foods into your diet portfolio. Don't think of the portfolio diet as a diet. Think of it as an investment in lower cholesterol.

That advice comes from David J.A. Jenkins, MD, and creator of the portfolio diet. The University of Toronto nutrition expert prefers to call it, a dietary portfolio. Whatever he calls it, Jenkins and colleagues have shown that their portfolio diet plan cuts cholesterol in a similar manner as cholesterol-lowering drugs.

"We would like to see people do this on their own" says Jenkins. "The portfolio diet isn't designed as a weight loss diet. Its focus is on lowering cholesterol, but there's no reason why you can't incorporate the foods in the portfolio diet into a weight loss plan."

Putting Cholesterol-Lowering Securities in Your Diet Portfolio

When you invest in a retirement portfolio, you spread your money, across several different kinds of investments. The idea is to maximize your benefits while minimizing your risks.

The Portfolio diet calls for the same kind of investment in cholesterol lowering foods. Just as you wouldn't bet all your money on a single stock, Jenkins says you shouldn't bet your health on a single kind of healthy food.

He says, "We want people to look at the combinations of foods --." It is well recognized that as your cholesterol count goes up, so does your risk of heart disease. The safest way to lower cholesterol is by diet. But until recently, experts thought that most people couldn't significantly lower their cholesterol by diet alone.

Certain changes to the diet can lower cholesterol. Jenkins incorporated this into a palatable, tasty diet that includes soy, fiber, plant sterols, and nuts.

The portfolio diet recipe for lower cholesterol focuses on four kinds of food:

- ✓ The Portfolio diet substitutes soy-based foods for meat. "We are looking at soy-based meat substitutes such as soy burgers, soy hot dogs, and soy cold cuts," Jenkins says. "And we also used soy milk as a dairy substitute." For Thanksgiving, he suggests, one might replace turkey with "tofurkey."

- ✓ The Portfolio diet incorporates as much fiber as possible. Those on the portfolio diet take three daily servings of fiber (psyllium). Oats and barley replace other grains on this diet

- ✓ Although the Portfolio diet replaces butter and margarine with plant sterol-enriched margarines, most other researchers try to avoid these foods, instead substituting olive oil. The amount of Plant Sterols in these 'enriched margarines' is minimal, and there is still the problem of the margarine itself. It is much better to take a plant sterols dietary supplement.

✓ The portfolio diet includes nuts. Study participants ate a handful of almonds every day. Obviously other tree nuts also help reduce cholesterol and are high in healthy fats.

As with many diets, the foods in the Portfolio diet are available in supermarkets and your corner store. Some of the healthy items from atypical day on the portfolio diet include:

☑ Breakfast. Soy milk, oat-bran cereal with chopped fruit and almonds, oatmeal bread

☑ Lunch. Soy cold cuts, oat-bran bread, bean soup, and fruit

☑ Dinner. Vegetables, tofu, fruit, and almonds

☑ Snacks. Nuts, yogurt, and soy milk thickened with psyllium powder

Jenkins and colleagues have shown that people who religiously follow their portfolio diet can lower their cholesterol. He claims a 20% reduction in the 'bad' LDL cholesterol after six months in 33% of his participants, which is quite good. 31% of participants had a 15% reduction in LDL cholesterol, but 35% of participants failed to lower their cholesterol at all. The foods in the portfolio diet can be added to almost any healthy diet as we have shown in various chapters of this book.

Body for Life Diet

What Is It?

As I have mentioned in various parts of this book, there are many different approaches to healthy diets. Some are more radical than others, and some more successful than others. In the end, for the most part, the ones I will present in this book are not harmful to your health, and if followed will be beneficial.

One of these is the Body-for-Life Diet that is an intense exercise, and nutrition program based on the principle that you are more likely to stick to a diet and workout if you quickly see results. Bill Phillips developed this diet.

The program is challenging. It involves training with weights for 45 minutes 3 days a week, then alternating with aerobic exercise for at least 20 minutes 3 days a week

The diet involves eating 6 small meals each day for 6 days a week, drawing from a list of healthy foods such as vegetables, brown rice, poultry, and fish. On the seventh day, you rest - you are free to eat anything you want and take a day off from the rigorous workout.

As with most popularized diets, you'll see before-and-after photos of people who went from flabby to very trim and fit. Take these with a grain of salt—electronic photo modifications are very good. The key, of course, is that strenuous exercise, even if you weren't also dieting, would significantly improve your body.

What You Can Eat

The good news is that Body-for-Life requires you eat. The key is grazing not gorging. The program requires you to eat six moderate-sized meals a day.

Each meal consists of:

- ☑ A fist-sized portion of protein - lean poultry, tofu, fish, cottage cheese, or egg whites.
- ☑ A fist-sized portion of carbohydrates such as potatoes or brown rice.
- ☑ You must also eat at least two portions of vegetables
- ☑ Drink 10 glasses of water each day.
- ☑ Nutritional supplements (sold by another company that Phillips founded)
- ☑ A tablespoon or two of healthy oil, such as flaxseed, round out the diet

The diet breaks down to about 40%-50% protein, the same for carbohydrates, and very little fat. Whereas a traditional weight-loss diet is usually 60% carbohydrates, 20-25% protein, and 20-25% fat.

Some of the suggested foods from the Body-for-Life diet appear appropriate and healthy such as proteins, which include chicken breast, turkey breast, swordfish, tuna, salmon, haddock, egg whites, and non-fat cottage cheese.

Carbohydrates include sweet potato, yam, baked potato, pumpkin, squash, whole grain pasta, steamed brown rice, steamed wild rice, oatmeal, beans, barley, corn, melon, apples; oranges, strawberries, fat-free yogurt, and whole-grain bread.

Vegetables include asparagus, broccoli, cauliflower, green beans, lettuce, carrot, green pepper, mushroom, tomato, peas, spinach, Brussels sprouts, artichoke, celery, cabbage, zucchini, cucumber, and onion.

How It Works

Bottom line: *You eat fewer calories and you burn more calories in exercise.*

The foods on Body-for-Life's authorized list tend to be lower in calories than standard American fare. By eating fist-sized portions, you are sure to consume fewer calories, even if you are eating six meals a day.

Also, the intense weight lifting will build muscle, which lifts your metabolic rate all day. By exercising strenuously six days a week, eventually you'll burn more calories around the clock.

What the Experts Say

Obviously this diet can be effective if you follow it closely, but it may require too much exercise for most people.

"There's an element of truth and an element of science and a lot of hype to this program," says fitness expert Steven N. Blair PED, Director of Research at the renowned Cooper Institute in Dallas.

Unfortunately, fewer than 15% of adult Americans get as much exercise as the recommended three 10-minute walks a day and consequently it is not likely to be a cure all for the burgeoning obesity problem.

Ornish Diet

The Ornish Diet, unlike many other diet books that make big promises, *Eat More, Weigh Less*, by Dean Ornish, MD, soft-pedals the health claims for this diet for the masses. It is adapted from his regimen, to reverse heart disease. Ornish is well known in the medical community because of his success in reversing blockages to the heart, once thought impossible without surgery, or drugs.

Ornish's explanations are simple and well supported. His main point is that eating a high-fiber, low-fat, vegetarian diet will not only help you become healthy and stay healthy, it will also help you lose weight.

According to Ornish, this is accomplished, by a combination of diet, and exercise that allows the body's fat burning mechanism to work most effectively.

The Ornish Diet - What You Can Eat

The Ornish says that we will find success not by restricting calories, but by watching the ones we eat. He breaks this down into foods that should be eaten all of the time, some of the time, and none of the time.

The following can be eaten whenever you are hungry, until you are full: beans and legumes, fruits -- anything from apples to watermelon, from raspberries to pineapples, grains, and vegetables.

These should be eaten in moderation:

- ☑ Nonfat dairy products -- skim milk, nonfat yogurt, nonfat cheeses, nonfat sour cream, and egg whites

- ☑ Nonfat or very low-fat commercially available products --from Life Choice frozen dinners to Haagen-Dazs frozen yogurt bars and Entenmann's fat-free desserts (if sugar is among the first few ingredients listed, put it back on the shelf)

These should always be avoided:

- ☑ Meat of all kinds -- red and white, fish, and fowl (if you can't give up meat all together, you should at least eat as little as possible per month)
- ☑ Oils and oil-containing products, such as margarine and most salad dressings
- ☑ Avocados (I do not agree with him here-in moderation, this is good fat)
- ☑ Olives

☑ Nuts and seeds (I do not agree with him here-these are good food)

☑ Dairy products (other than the nonfat ones above)

☑ Sugar and simple sugar derivatives -- honey, molasses, corn syrup, and high-fructose syrup

☑ Alcohol

☑ Anything commercially prepared that has more than two grams of fat per serving

That's it. If you stick to his plan, you will meet Ornish's recommendation of less than 10% of your calories from fat without the need to count fat grams or calories. Ornish suggests eating a lot of little meals, because this diet makes you feel hungry more often. You will feel full faster, and you'll eat more food without increasing the number of calories.

Ornish's regimen is more than mere diet he claims. He is a stickler about incorporating at least 30 minutes of moderate exercise a day, or an hour three times a week and using some kind of stress management technique, which might include meditation, massage, psychotherapy, or yoga.

How It Works

Ornish suggests that our metabolism was set back in Fred Flintstone's era, when we didn't know where our next meal was coming from and there were times when little food was available. The body naturally wanted to hang onto all the energy it could and would try to store any extra energy as fat. Nowadays, most of us have almost continuous access to food, but our bodies haven't adapted to this new way of living.

Because the rate at which you are burning calories can decrease when you consume fewer calories, you may hit a plateau soon after you began a new, lower-calorie diet. For most of us, the pounds seem to melt away for a delightful week or two, but then that scale doesn't budge. Our weight stays the same, sometimes for a week, sometimes much longer.

But Ornish argues that with this eat-all-you-want, eat-as-often-as-you-are-hungry routine, your metabolism stays the same, or better yet, even increases. The high-fiber content also slows down the absorption of food into the digestive system, so you feel full longer with small portions, than you would eating calorie-restricted small portions. The complex carbohydrates don't cause your blood sugar, the level of glucose in the blood, to yo-yo. It remains more stable, and so do you.

Ornish gives more than a passing nod to physical activity, encouraging long, slow exercise that uses body fat as fuel. Moderate exercise done on a regular basis revs up your resting metabolism, while some have suggested that short periods of intense exercise decrease metabolism.

Although he doesn't claim that meditation will make the pounds dissolve, his regimen incorporates it as a way of quieting your mind, increasing self-awareness, and coping with stress. He calls it food for the soul. "When your soul is fed, you have less need to overeat," he writes in *Eat More, Weigh Less*. "When you directly experience the fullness of life, then you have less need to fill the void with food."

Mostly, Ornish gets kudos from the medical community for his highly restricted diet and healthy lifestyle routine. His documented studies showing a reversal of coronary blockage are indeed impressive.

Neal Barnard, MD, president of the Physicians Committee for Responsible Medicine, says, "His diet is one of the only popular diet plans that is firmly rooted in science. It not only brings weight loss without counting calories, but it also brings good overall health. It reverses heart disease, cuts the risk of cancer, makes diabetes and hypertension more manageable, and sometimes even makes them go away."

The drawback is that the plan requires learning completely new eating habits, which many consider drastic. Barnard, the author of *Food for Life* and several other books on health, adds, "But after the first week or two, the plan becomes self-rewarding, because the weight loss is virtually automatic. People have better energy and they just want to stick to it."

On the other hand, Robert H. Eckel, MD, chair of the nutrition committee of the American Heart Association and a professor at the University of Colorado Health Sciences Center, is doubtful. He suggests that only the most committed will stick to Ornish's routine: "Many people get tired of eating food with such a low fat content."

Frank Hu, MD, PhD, assistant professor of medicine at the Harvard School of Public Health, is critical of how severely fat is limited on the diet" The data from numerous studies show that it is the type of fat, rather than the total amount, which is related to cardiovascular health," he says. "Polyunsaturated and monounsaturated oils actually protect against cardiovascular incidents, but Ornish doesn't distinguish the good fats from the bad fats (which I also think is a good thing to differentiate) – such as trans fats, which come from margarine sticks and cookies and crackers, and animal fats."

For example, Hu says, Ornish advocates limiting the consumption of fish and nuts, and Hu adds, "There is strong evidence that the fat in them is protective against coronary heart disease in both epidemiological studies and clinical trials."

The recommendation to eat smaller, more frequent meals requires that dieters change their eating schedules, which could be difficult for some but a very effective way to diet, and keep healthy. This same theory, "eat like a chicken not a tiger". His plan has what it takes to lose weight and keep it off, and receives high marks from nutrition experts.

Vegetarian Diet

In this book we have discussed a variety of dietary programs, all of which are geared to a healthier lifestyle, or to healing some specific disease. We have seen that the constituents of diets that are healthy, and encourage a longer more enjoyable life, involve a large quantity of complex carbohydrates including fresh and steamed vegetables, legumes, nuts, soy derivatives, whole grains, and fruits.

None of these diets recommend animal protein (meat) as a basis. Diets that do emphasize high protein diets with meat as a basis are fraught with problems, and those that follow them usually end up with renal problems and liver problems and a host of other medical problems.

I realize that a great portion of this country and others have invested a great deal socially and economically in the production, distribution, marketing and consumption of meat, and its byproducts.

For those involved in this "machine", it is nearly impossible to even think of the possibility of eliminating meat from their diet. Culturally, many have 'grown up' with meat as a substantial constituent in their diet. It has been drummed into their head that they will not live if they do not eat meat. They are not only mistaken– they are badly mistaken.

The fact that the majority of one of the most populous nations in the world are all vegetarian is just one interesting statistic to the overabundance of facts and figures that support a change to a meatless diet, from a medical and philosophical basis.

Many tomes have been written on this topic, and I will not attempt to replicate the vast information available. What I will do here is outline some of the interesting facts with a scientific basis that supports the medical and philosophical change to a meatless diet - for example, a vegetarian diet.

Study Data on the Health Benefits of a Vegetarian Diet

In the United States, the total direct medical costs attributable to meat consumption were estimated at between $30-60 billion a year, based the significantly more common cases of obesity, hypertension, gallstones, cancer, heart disease, diabetes, and food borne illness among omnivores compared with those who are vegetarians.

A large body of scientific research shows eating a diet of legumes, whole grains, nuts, fruits, and vegetables, while avoiding meat and high-fat animal products; when combined with regular exercise; is directly linked to lower blood pressure, and lower blood cholesterol levels, as well as a reduction in obesity, cancer, stroke, diabetes, heart disease, and mortality.

A vegetarian diet is different from an omnivorous diet by its content of dry beans and lentils, replacing meat and fish, as the major source of protein. There are all kinds of beans you can choose from - lima, kidney, soybeans, cranberry, pinto, navy, garbanzo, black-eyed peas, and Great Northern. These can be added to soups or stews, served with rice, and served as salads, or in a variety of casseroles.

Tofu, or soy bean curd, can be used in dips and spreads. It can be served with stir-fried vegetables, or pasta. Soy protein contains isoflavones that act as phytoestrogens and inhibit tumor growth, decrease the risk of blood clots, diminish bone loss, and lower blood cholesterol levels. These benefits clearly translate into a lower risk of cancer, heart disease, osteoporosis, and stroke.

Cancer

A 1997 report published by the World Cancer Research Fund recommended we could lower our risk of cancer by selecting mainly plant-based diets rich in a variety of fruits, and vegetables, legumes, and a minimal amount of processed starchy staple foods, as well as by limiting the intake of cured, smoked, and grilled meats and fish. When meats are prepared in this manner the amount of polycyclic aromatic hydrocarbons and heterocyclic amines, which are both known carcinogens, is reduced.

There have been more than 200 studies, which have revealed regularly eating fruits, and vegetables provide a great deal of protection against cancer. Those eating a diet consistently high in fruits and vegetables cut their risk of cancer in half, especially for epithelial cancers. Other cancers saw a reduced risk of 20%-50% in those who had diets high in whole grains compared to those with a lower intake.

More than three-dozen foods have been identified as possessing cancer - protective properties. These include cruciferous vegetables, such as Brussels sprouts, broccoli, cabbage, and cauliflower; cilantro, carrots, dill, celery, caraway, and parsley; as well as other fruits and vegetables such as tomatoes, citrus, cucumber, cantaloupe, berries, and grapes; beans.

Whole grains such as oats, brown rice, and whole wheat; many nuts, flaxseed, and a variety of seasoning herbs such as garlic, onions, scallions, chives, turmeric, ginger, thyme, rosemary, oregano, sage, and basil, are also included.

These foods and herbs contain a number of cancer protective phytochemicals such as flavonoids, carotenoids, isothiocyanates, glucarates, liminoids, curcumins, saponins, tocotrienols, phytosterols, phthalides, and sulfide compounds.

These beneficial compounds stimulate the immune system, as well as change metabolic pathways that are associated with the development of cancer. They are also an incredibly powerful antioxidant.

Heart Disease Diet

The consumption of fruits and vegetables reduces the risk of ischemic heart disease. A recently conducted survey of 47,000 Italians found those with the highest percentile of vegetable consumption had a 21% reduced risk of myocardial infarction, and an 11% reduced risk angina, compared with those in the lowest percentile of vegetable consumption.

A British study found that daily consumption of fresh fruit was directly linked to a 24% reduction in mortality from heart disease, and a 32% reduction in death from cerebrovascular disease, compared to those who rarely eat fruit. The consumption of raw salad saw a 26% reduction in mortality from heart disease.

In another study of lifelong vegetarians (those who eat no eggs or dairy products) there was a 57% lower incidence of coronary heart disease compared to those who ate meat. Healthy volunteers who consumed a vegetarian diet rich in green, leafy vegetables, and other low-calorie vegetables (cucumbers, tomatoes, carrots, corn, celery, peas, green beans, etc.), fruits, and nuts, saw a significant reduction in bad cholesterol, and triglycerides with an increase in good cholesterol, in just 2 weeks.

Various factors exist in fruits, and vegetables that have the potential to offer protection against cardiovascular disease. These factors include dietary fiber, folic acid, potassium, carotenoids, phytosterols, magnesium, flavonoids, and other polyphenol antioxidants.

Typically, vegetarian diets are also lower in saturated fat, and cholesterol. Vegetarians generally have lower blood cholesterol levels. Plant diets rich in soluble fiber are helpful in lowering serum cholesterol levels.

The many flavonoids in fruits, vegetables, whole grains, and nuts have ample biological properties that lower the risk of heart disease. Flavonoids are some of the most potent antioxidants.

They protect LDL cholesterol from oxidation, and they inhibit the forming of blood clots. They also have anti-inflammatory action. European studies showed those with the highest consumption of flavonoids had a 70% lower risk of stroke, and a 60% lower mortality rate from heart disease than those who consumed none or few flavonoids.

The yellow, orange, and red carotenoids in fruits and vegetables are powerful antioxidants that can quench free radicals and protect against cholesterol oxidation. Those with high levels of serum carotenoids have a reduced risk of heart disease.

The recent EURAMIC study saw a 48% lower risk of myocardial infarction in men with a high intake of lycopene (the red pigment in pink grapefruit, tomatoes, and watermelon) compared to those with a low intake of lycopene.

Stroke and Diabetes Diet

Data from two studies supports strong relationship between the consumption of fruits and vegetables and a reduction in the risk of ischemic stroke. The study found that cruciferous and green leafy vegetables and citrus fruits offered the most protection.

Data from the NHANES study showed that those who ate fruits and vegetables at least three times a day had

- A 27% lower incidence of stroke
- A 27% lower cardiovascular disease mortality
- A 42% lower stroke mortality
- A 15% lower all-cause mortality

compared with those who ate fruits and vegetables one times a day or less.

In the Adventist Health Study, non-vegetarians had a 20-30% higher risk of fatal stroke than those who are vegetarians. Data from population studies and human trials provides evidence that vegetarian dietary patterns lower blood pressure.

A number of studies have shown that a higher consumption of whole grains and nuts is associated with lower rates of diabetes. In one large study, eating fruits and vegetables was found to be inversely associated with the incidence of diabetes, particularly among women.

Men and women who, seldom or never, eat fruits or green leafy vegetables had higher HbA levels, than those who frequently consumed fruits and green leafy vegetables. An increased consumption of fruits and vegetables has been show to contribute to the prevention of diabetes.

French Diet

The French feast on rich food, yet they stay slim. How do they do it? Flaky croissants, plump snails and frogs' legs swimming in butter, triple-fat cheese, melt-in-your mouth foe gras (goose or duck liver) and clouds of chocolate mousse. For centuries, the French living in north and central France has feasted on such guilty pleasures. Yet, on the streets of Paris, most women appear enviably slim.

In fact, despite their rich diet, the French generally are slimmer than Americans. According to the Institut National de la Sante et la Recherché Medicale in Paris (the equivalent to the National Institutes of Health), just 8% of the French qualify as obese, compared to 33% of Americans.

How They Do It

How do the French do it? It's more than good genes – and Americans may well want to follow their lead. How? The French tend to snack less and savor their meals more slowly -- which could lead to eating less food overall.

The eating patterns of the French offer significant clues to their healthfulness. For one, they traditionally don't take lunch lightly. In a study that tracked the eating habits of 50 blue-collar workers in Paris and Boston, the French participants consumed 60% of their day's calories before 2 p.m., followed later by a small dinner, so they were less likely to sleep on a major calorie cushion.

Second, the study found that the French participants didn't snack, defined as consuming one to two between-meal foods, such as a handful of peanuts and a glass of orange juice. "The French ate less than one snack a day.

Here in the U.S., we have about three snacks a day," says lead researcher. R. Curtis Ellison, MD, professor of preventive medicine, and epidemiology at Boston University School of Medicine. Like Americans, the French traditionally consume three meals a day. But that's where the similarity ends.

For the French, lunch and dinner are the most structured meals, consisting of a starter, such as crudités raw vegetables followed by a main course, a salad, the cheese course, and perhaps dessert. Their substantial lunch and dinner often usurps the need for a snack.

As a result, "snacking is simply not part of the culture," says Annie Jacquet-Bentley, a Parisian restaurant consultant currently based in Birchrunville, Pa. Her eating habits remain fiercely snack-free despite having lived in the snack-filled U.S. for more than 20 years.

Meals in France traditionally are regarded as experiences to be savored -- sanctimonious time-outs that a snack can otherwise spoil. "Even if the French don't have a lot of time, they will sit down and have a two- or three-course meal," Jacquet-Bentley says. "Food is a life pleasure, and it's meant to be enjoyed. For both lunch and dinner, people tend not to rush if they can help it."

Granted, snacking in French cities like Paris is gaining ground -- the Paris Metro, for example, recently installed vending machines in several stations. Still, many French find the practice distasteful. According to the European Snack Food Association, 81% of French consumers surveyed think that eating between meals can be a problem or is clearly unhealthy.

America the Snack Attack Nation

On the other hand, in the U.S., snacking is a $30 billion industry that has increased 33% since 1988, according to the U.S. Snack Food Association, with high-fat, high-calorie options, such as pork rinds, cheese, and corn snacks, leading sales.

It seems downright un-American not to snack. Still, according to a 1998 survey conducted by the Calorie Control Council in Atlanta, GA, 43% of adult Americans blame snacking as the reason they can't maintain their desired weight.

"Snacking can be detrimental to weight loss because you're confronting food more often," says Karen Miller-Kovach, MS, RD, chief scientist at Weight Watchers International, in which case, it's often harder to stop eating once you've started.

Snacking also can be fattening because it contributes to total calorie consumption. According to a 1993 study published in the medical journal Appetite, which managed to find 273 obese French women, those in the study who snacked (60%) ate more at meals and between meals than those who didn't.

"The less often you eat, the fewer calories you consume," says David Levitsky, PhD, professor of nutritional sciences at Cornell University in Ithaca, N.Y., who has conducted numerous studies on snacking. According to Levitsky, when people are allowed snacks, they may eat as much at their next meal as if they didn't snack. All told, snackers tend to consume more total calories than nonsnackers, Levitsky says.

Taming the Snacking Tiger

On the other hand, snacking doesn't have to be all bad. It may even help you lose weight if you snack judiciously or have frequent, smaller meals throughout the day -- as long as they're nutritious. "

Having a regular pattern of snacks can be an effective strategy to keep hunger at bay so you don't overeat at the next meal," Miller-Kovach says. However, snacking is a dieting strategy that works for some people and not for others. "If you're going to snack, you need to be a planner," Miller-Kovach says. She offers three tips to fit snacking into your diet without blowing your calorie budget:

1. **Be prepared:** Don't let a snack attack take you by surprise. For example, to resist calorie-laden vending machine fare, have healthy, satisfying snack foods on hand, such as nonfat yogurt, fresh fruit (apples, oranges, or bananas), dried fruit (raisins), rice cakes, animal crackers, low-cal beverages, (herbal tea, flavored seltzer, diet hot chocolate), and packets of unflavored instant oatmeal.

In general, foods rich in calcium, such as low-fat or nonfat yogurt; iron, such as lentil soup; or fiber, such as whole-grain crackers, are good snacking choices because they contain nutrients lacking in many American women's diets. If you have trouble stopping at one serving, buy single-serving containers, says Fran Grossman, MS, RD, a nutritionist at Mount Sinai Medical Center in New York City.

2. **Get it right:** Snacks have a way of working themselves into your day. To avoid snacking amnesia (did I eat that?), write down the snacks you eat in a food diary. Even better, try reverse journaling, suggests Miller-Kovach. Record the snacks you plan to consume then check off each after you've eaten it. (You can use this weight loss strategy for meals, too.)

3. **Personalize your snacking choices:** To make sure your snack hits the spot, "find your personal preference in terms of what satisfies you," Miller-Kovach says. For example, if you tend to like crunchy snacks, stock your desk drawer with an apple or a tiny box of animal crackers. If you crave creaminess, try fat free yogurt, low-fat yogurt, low-fat vanilla pudding, or low-fat chocolate pudding. Seeking something salty? Opt for fat-free pretzels. Something sweet? Go for sorbet or a frozen yogurt pop.

If you'd rather do like the French and avoid snacking, then you should eat more at meals and have something to drink -- water or a diet beverage -- should a snack attack hit. If that doesn't work, and the chocolate bar or corn chips still call your name, go ahead and press that vending machine button. But whatever you do, don't gobble guiltily. Instead, do like the French when it comes to eating in general.

Eating Well for Optimum Health

The Weil's Approach

What It Is

There's no hocus-pocus here, no magic, and no quick weight-loss promises from the controversial wellness guru Andrew Weil, MD. Weil sums up his philosophy in just four words: "Eat less, exercise more." Weil, the author of several best-sellers, including the latest, *Eating Well for Optimum Health*, urges everyone to be sensible when it comes to their eating habits, which is more an Eastern trait than a Western trait. Weil concentrates on Eastern philosophy in a number of his tomes.

What we eat directly influences our health, and not just a little bit, but in a big way. However, Andrew Weil does warn that diet is only one aspect of our lifestyle; just as lifestyle is only one variable in the mix of factors that determine whether we are blessed with well being, or whether we feel out of sorts.

That said, Weil claims that diet can positively impact numerous health concerns, from allergies to body odor, from ear infections to irritable bowel syndrome, from arthritis to sinusitis, and it can also make it easy to control our weight. He, like many, urges readers not to seek solutions promising quick weight loss. Instead, he agrees with most nutritionists to set a realistic goal, of a maximum weight loss of one to two pounds a week.

According to Weil, the science is straightforward. Successful weight loss can be accomplished by correctly balancing the amount and type of food we eat. The key is to determine the kinds of foods to put on your plate.

What You Can Eat On the Weil Diet

Weil's approach is very similar to the Mediterranean Diet. One of the major differences that should be noted is that the Mediterranean diet does include red meat where as Weil is also not a fan of meat. Weil's diet plan breaks down the three food groups this way:

1. Carbohydrates

Weil also says that carbohydrates should make up 50-60% of your calorie intake. The majority should be from complex carbohydrates. Good carbs include fruit, grains (such as stone-ground whole-wheat bread) and pulses.

2. Fats

Weil allows up to 30% of calories can come from monounsaturated fats.

3. Protein

Weil limits protein in his diet to 10-20% of the diet and substitutes vegetable proteins for animal ones as often as possible.

How It Works

Weil does not give a lot of scientific mumbo jumbo in his book. Instead, he presents a basic primer in human nutrition and describes how the body gets energy from food.

Weil is critical of the high-protein diets that send us into the altered state of ketosis, as it may be detrimental to our health over the long term according to Weil. The best carbohydrates are unrefined grains and vegetables –these are said to have a low glycemic index.

Second, fats and oils are more concentrated sources of energy than carbohydrates, and are converted into glucose to be used by the body. Although fat has a bad name in today's collective health consciousness, some fat is essential.

Weil cites exercise as a critical component of his program, but has little to say about the subject other than that regular exercise increases caloric output and in time can change the basic weight-loss equation in your favor, and help you keep off the pounds over the long term.

What the Experts Say

Nutrition experts support Weil's diet as a common-sense approach that is based on well-accepted nutritional principles. The experts agree, his plan is a healthy one, because in general people who eat similar diets tend to be healthier than those who don't.

Michael Janson, MD, past president of the American Preventive Medical Association and the author of Dr. Janson's New Vitamin Revolution and the American Dietetic Association (ADA) also gives Weil's diet a nod of approval. Spokeswoman for the ADA and an associate professor of nutrition at Georgia State University in Atlanta,

Food For Thought

Among the array of popular diet writers, Weil recommends a particularly holistic approach. This means that dieters need to watch what they eat, while also considering the level of stress in their lives, the amount of exercise they do, and other factors.

It is a good practical plan for those willing to follow the guidelines. For those seeking a list of rigid "do's and don'ts" or easy-to-follow formulas, this plan may prove challenging. In addition, those who are used to diets high in dairy and red meat may find this diet unsatisfying.

CHAPTER 15

FAST FOOD DANGERS

Diseases such as arthritis, diabetes and cardiovascular complications have all been linked to eating too much fast food.

The hectic pace of life today, with long days at work, shorter lunch breaks, and later hours, many people have resorted to fast food restaurants - they are convenient and cheap.

Unfortunately, there's nothing healthy about eating this type of food, especially when it is consumed in excess. It can damage your health and result in diseases such as heart disease, obesity, and respiratory conditions, to name just a few.

According to one study, U.S. researchers found that those people who live in neighborhoods that have many fast food restaurants are much more likely to suffer a stroke.

University of London scientists recommend you decrease the amount of processed foods you eat to prevent obesity-related conditions. They suggest eating more fruits and vegetables, which contain antioxidants that help prevent to prevent disease

Dr McCulloch, director of the Mental Health Foundation, recommends a balanced diet with only the occasional eating of fast food restaurants and processed foods to reduce likelihood of problems.

In 2003, The Center for Disease Control and Prevention reported that, in the year 2000 - 1 out of 3 kids born in America will develop type 2-diabetes. Diabetes is the sixth-highest cause of death in America.

The life of a 10-year-old child with type II diabetes will be 20 to 25 years shorter than that of a healthy child. Diabetes can also lead to strokes, heart attacks, kidney failure, blindness, and nerve damage in the lower legs, which can cause an amputation. There are 82,000 of these amputations every year.

Fast Food Causes Obesity

The fast food industry adds every chemical that they can legally get away, which is designed to addict people to their food. Did you know if you eat fast food and you stop eating it, you would actually go through withdrawal symptoms? It's like a drug.

In addition, the preservatives are so high in these fast food burgers that the product doesn't break down. Fast food has been linked to increase obesity in adults and children. Obesity has reached epidemic proportions in America, especially in children. Here are some startling statistics to consider:

- ☑ 65% of American adults are overweight
- ☑ 30% of Americans are obese
- ☑ In the last 20 years, the rate of obesity has doubled in children and tripled in teens.
- ☑ According to the American Obesity Association, 127 million Americans are overweight, 60 million Americans are obese, and 9 million are "morbidly obese," which means they weigh more than 100 pounds more than they should.
- ☑ As of September 2004, 9 million American kids between the ages of 6 and 18 were obese.

Fast Food Causes Obesity and Obesity Kills

This year, obesity-related illnesses will kill around 400,000 Americans, which is almost the same number as smoking. Americans aren't just supersizing their fast food meal, they're supersizing their coffins.

Illnesses related to obesity include:

- ☑ High blood pressure
- ☑ High cholesterol
- ☑ Strokes
- ☑ Heart disease
- ☑ Colon cancer
- ☑ Breast Cancer
- ☑ Gout
- ☑ Asthma

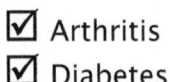

☑ Arthritis
☑ Diabetes

10 Dangerous Diseases caused by Steady Eating of Fast Food

1. Heart Disease

Heart disease is one of the most common diseases that is the result of eating too much fast food. When you have large amounts of body fat it often leads to high levels of LDL cholesterol, and low levels of HDL. Both of these factors can increase your risk of heart disease, which is the biggest cause of death around the world.

2. Type-2 Diabetes

Type-2 diabetes is related to obesity. Those who suffer from type-2 diabetes can't produce adequate insulin to convert sugar to energy. This is the result of a malfunctioning pancreas. The sugar ends up transported into the blood where it causes relentless damage to the body.

3. Dyslipidemia

This is a group of diseases characterized by an abnormal concentration of blood lipid levels. It occurs when the levels of bad cholesterol (LDL) and triglycerides are abnormally high. Most doctors feel that the development of these diseases is directly tied to weight gain.

4. Polycystic Ovary Syndrome

Overweight women are at greater risk of developing polycystic ovary syndrome. It is also a major cause of infertility in women of childbearing age. It leads to irregular menstrual cycles and increased hair growth.

5. Sleep Apnea

Sleep apnea is linked to obesity and is characterized by a person who stops breathing during their sleep.

6. Arthritis

While the relationship between obesity and arthritis is blurred, there is an important connection between uric acid levels and body weight. In addition, weight gain adds an unhealthy load on your joints.

7. Blount Disease

Obesity is dangerous for growing children. This condition develops when there is too much weight on the growing bones in the lower body, which can cause a growth that is abnormal.

8. Respiratory Problems

Being overweight puts more stress on the heart, and it also makes the lungs work harder to get more oxygen. When you have high bad cholesterol levels, it hinders oxygen from moving through the body easily. Obese people also suffer from asthma.

9. Liver Damage

Sometimes the body has trouble digesting fatty foods, and the fat can accumulate around the liver. This condition can lead to scarring and inflammation of the liver, and can lead to permanent damage.

10. Stroke

Strokes are caused when arteries are blocked that supply blood to the brain. When blood and oxygen are not able to reach the brain then the cells begin to die, which cause permanent brain damage. These blockages are seen more often in overweight people because they are more likely to have high cholesterol and high blood pressure.

You Find Fast Food Everywhere

The rise of the fast food industry plays a significant role in why our country is plagued with obesity. Fast food is everywhere – it's in the schools, in the bus stations, in cities, in small towns, at the shopping malls, at the airport, and it's even in hospitals!

There are 31,000 McDonald's worldwide – almost 14,000 of them are in the U.S.

People are Eating Way too Much Fast Food

☑ Fast food has become cheaper and easier to buy.

☑ In 2004, Americans spent $124 billion dollars on fast food.

☑ In 2004, The American Journal of Preventive Medicine published a study showing that the percentage of fast food calories in the American diet has increased from 3% to 12% over the last 20 years.

☑ It was around the 1980's when fast food culture was introduced to other countries around the world.

☑ In countries like Japan and China, people have abandoned traditional healthy diets in favor of fast food. As a result, their rate of obesity and other diseases has skyrocketed.

☑ Fast food companies encourage the consumer to eat more by supplying over-sized burgers, and extra-large servings of fries, and buckets of soda.

☑ The Double Gulp soda at your local 7-11 holds 64 ounces of soda - that's a whopping half-gallon! It contains the equivalent of 48 teaspoons of sugar.

☑ A typical hamburger at a fast food restaurant weighs 6 ounces. In 1957, it weighed only 1 ounce.

☑ The average meal at a McDonald's has 1,550 calories.

Fast Food is Bad for Us

☑ We're eating more food that is not nutritious.

☑ Most fast-food meals are high in fat, high in sugar, high in calories, high in starch, high in salt, and low in fiber and nutrients.

☑ Because fast food lacks nutrients, after we eat it we're not satisfied. That makes us hungry for more soon after.

Why Our Kids are at a Major Risk

☑ Our children are exposed to an ambush of advertising for fast food.

☑ Fast food chains spend more than $3 billion every year on TV advertising.

☑ They deliberately campaign to kids, so they become life-long customers. These are known as cradle-grave advertising strategies.

☑ Researchers have found that children can often recognize a company logo, like the Golden Arches before they can even recognize their own name.

☑ In one year, the typical American child watches more that 40,000 TV commercials. Around 20,000 of these ads are for junk food fast food, candy, soda, and breakfast cereals.

☑ Your child sees a junk food ad every 5 minutes when they are watching TV.

☑ To motivate kids to eat fast food companies like McDonald's have Happy Meals with free toys. McDonald's gives away more than 1.5 billion toys every year.

☑ Almost 1 out of every 3 new toys given to American kids each year is from McDonald's or another fast food restaurant.

In order to fight these intended advertising strategies, it is critical that we educate our children on healthy eating habits that are fun and easy. By teaching our children how bad fast food is and how to eat healthier, we are empowering them to make the right choices.

There are lots of healthy alternatives that can satisfy your cravings, but still deliver the vitamins and nutrients your body needs

CHAPTER 16

WEIGHT LOSS

Are you really overweight? Of course, there are a lot of people who feel that their body type is too big, i.e., being overweight.

This can be from watching commercials of models that have bulimia, and starve themselves to become the shape that they are, and expected to be for the magazine covers that they adorn. There are a small minority of Caucasians, many Orientals, and some tribes of Blacks that are genetically very thin.

These are the lucky ones to the rest of us that have to 'watch what we eat'. For some the genetic predisposition is to be very heavy. Others are just average, but can make us very heavy by our learned habits of eating the wrong things and overeating and not exercising.

But, first things first. Are you really overweight? There is a scientific way of determining this. It is called the BMI, or Body Mass Index. This is a good way of determining if the average muscled individual with normal bone structure is or isn't overweight. The exceptions are the bulked up body builders of the world and those athletes that put significant stress on their bone structure so as to abnormally increase the weight of the bones. (These athletes are usually not overweight anyway!!)

Here goes:

1. Convert your weight to pounds and multiply by 703.
2. Convert your height to inches and multiply by itself.
3. Divide the answer to #1 by the answer to #2.

If your BMI score is:

Under 25, you have normal weight.
Between 25 & 29, you are overweight.
At or over 30, you are considered obese.

The New Weight Loss

Losing weight and maintaining a normal weight is an important role for many people. That's the finding of many surveys, which show that 63.1% of adults in the U.S. were either overweight or obese and the more recent statistics indicate even higher percentages in North American cities.

That was even an increase from the previous year. Another survey found that 36.6% of Americans are overweight and 26.5% obese. Unfortunately, too many people spend countless hours and dollars trying to lose weight and do not change their approach to weight loss for the long term, which is the most important thing to do.

The *Gallup–Healthways Well–Being Index* based on telephone interviews with 673,000 adults in January 2008 to December 2009 found that:

☑ Obese Americans exercise less than normal weight people. Obese people are less likely than people in every other weight category (overweight, normal weight, underweight) to have eaten five servings of fruits and vegetables, on at least three days of the past seven.

☑ Obese Americans also are less likely to say they ate healthy "all day yesterday."

☑ 71.6% of normal-weight people were found to eat the recommended five servings of fruits three to seven days per week, obese people much less.

People who are obese are far more likely to report being diagnosed with high blood pressure, high cholesterol, diabetes, or to have had a heart attack.

The survey found that:

☑ Of people with high blood pressure, 46.2% were obese

☑ Of people with high cholesterol, 36.8% were obese, 19.2% normal weight

☑ Of people with diabetes, 21.1% were obese, 5% normal weight

☑ Of depressed people, 23.3% were obese

The survey says that African-Americans in 2009 were among the most likely to be obese, at 36.2%, compared to the national average of 26.5%. The obesity rate among Hispanics, at 28.3%, is also higher than the national average. Asians are far less likely to be obese, with only 9.6% falling into that category.

The report concludes that obesity is still on the rise and that reversing this trend may require the involvement of communities, businesses, and governments.

By the World Health Organization's definition, adults are considered overweight if their body mass index (BMI) is 25-29.9, and obese if the BMI is 30 or more. The prevalence of obesity in Canada has progressed rapidly over the years.

The proportion of Canadian adults who are obese almost tripled in the last 15 years, from 5.6% in 1985 to 14.9% by 2000/2001. The case is even worse for males – their obesity rate is not only higher, but has also risen faster than their female counterpart.

In England, 16 % of women and 13% of men are obese. Being overweight means that there is excess fat, which is either visible or felt by the individual. Being obese means that the individual has gone well over the accepted limits of any national standard for body mass index.

Whether a person is the apple or pear shape, obesity is dangerous to many aspects of the human body. Certain shapes are more indicative of potential danger to the cardiovascular system.

Besides the heart, various other circulatory elements are at risk when a person is obese and all joints are at risk of having medical problems such as arthritis, ligament stain, etc.

Losing weight is never simple, and as one gets older it becomes more difficult. There are truly no easy solutions, no magic pills, and no fairy dust that will ever work at making people lose weight. There are allopathic and herbal combinations, which will help one's appetite.

There are herbal combinations that will help burn up fat such as Ayurvedic oils, which will help massage away fat and there are exercise programs, which will help to burn up excess fat.

Garcinia (Citrimax) is the bark of a tree that kills appetite if taken 30 minutes before a meal, and helps burn fat. It does NOT speed up the heart or tax the thyroid like Hoodia and various other herbal speed concoctions. Chromium picolinate (200 mg) helps the pancreas work properly and therefore, can help with weight control (and as a preventive for diabetes).

In the end, every dieter knows that overweight is not static, and without a successful diet they will not be able to permanently lose weight. You must eat fewer calories than your body burns, which will help weight loss.

Increasing caloric work, i.e.| through exercise also helps. Starvation/high protein no-carb (Atkins) diets do not work on a long-term basis and can be very detrimental to an individual. Although you may lose some weight initially, if you survive (remember Dr Atkins died from following his diet), but unless you then follow a rational and balanced diet, you will gain all those losses back, and then some (compensatory gain).

The basic principles of an appropriate weight loss diet include decreasing the total caloric intake that is derived from fat and decreasing the total fat intake. Basic in this diet is also increasing the fiber, and the foods that will help increase the burning of fat. The best formula for weight loss also includes a moderate amount of exercise. The total amount of exercise is not as important as the regularity of that exercise.

Studies have shown that with daily exercise not only maintains agility but an important psychological activation of the body necessary for weight loss is also activated. 20 minutes of any form of active exercise is an appropriate and desired end point in an appropriate weight loss program.

We are well aware of the fact that in the modern world with normal lives, nobody can adhere to any diet 100% of the time. But just because we cheat once in awhile doesn't mean we have to lose all that we gained in weight loss.

Consequently, there are substances that will 'eat up' excess fat that we may have consumed in a particular meal. These natural and chemical fat binders allow one to cheat once in a while, and not have significant problems with their cholesterol, such that the heart could be blocked at any instant, or a significant amount of fat would be restored into the liver.

Fat binders and cholesterol binding agents fall under several categories including colestipol Xenical and various amino polysaccharides derived from the exoskeleton of crustaceans that have the ability to absorb several times their own weight in fat.

These amino polysaccharides molecules are positively charged and therefore, attract the negatively charged carboxylic groups like fat, lipids, and bile. These cannot be reabsorbed, so they pass unchanged into the stool.

Focus on Thinking Differently to Lose Weight

Are you waiting until you've reached your goal weight to "think thin?" "Don't," say weight loss experts. The time to start thinking – and living – as a thinner healthier person is right now.

"Too often, people hold on to the belief that they can't think or act like a thin person until they reach their goal weight," says Linda Spangle, RN, MA, owner of Weight Loss for Life in Denver and author of *Life is Hard, Food is Easy: The 5-Step Plan to Overcome Emotional Eating and Lose Weight on Any Diet*. But staying trapped in your old, unhealthy mindset can sabotage the very behaviors you're trying so hard to change.

"I encourage people who are trying to lose weight to build an image of how they would not only look, but also how they would act and feel when they are thin," says Spangle.

For example, if you are a visual person, hang a favorite outfit where you can see it every day, then picture how well the outfit is going to fit you. If you're a movement-oriented person, picture how it would "feel" to slide easily past the empty seats in the theater row, or imagine the ease of fastening a seat belt in an airplane.

Pretend You Are Thin

Spangle teaches her clients to "pretend" they are thin and live as if that's true. When we pretend something is true, a new pattern of behavior will eventually evolve, says Spangle.

"Acting as if you have a skill or a feeling eventually contributes to it coming true," she says. "Public speakers are taught to address their audience as if they feel totally confident and have no stage fright whatsoever. Most speakers discover that after doing this even a few times, it becomes true."

In the same way, Spangle says, you don't have to wait until "someday" to have self-esteem. You can build your confidence and self-image by acting as if you already feel good about yourself (even if you don't). When you get dressed each day, look in the mirror and say, "I look great!" Then walk and talk as if you do.

"It doesn't matter if you're wearing a baggy dress and worn shoes," says Spangle. "Pretend! Imagine how you would talk to others, do your work projects, and raise your children if you truly felt great about yourself. Then live out of that internal picture, acting as if those things were true."

That doesn't mean you should pretend yourself right out of your need to develop more healthy habits. "Taking this approach doesn't mean you can put your head in the sand or ignore the realities of life," Spangle says. "It just helps you develop a new attitude about what's already there."

At the same time, it also gives you hope that things can get better. After a month or so, of living as if you are confident and strong about yourself, you will be amazed at how well you match this image.

Change Your Thinking

Another key to thinking and living like a thin person is to change your negative thought patterns.

"If you're struggling with your weight, it's important to examine your thinking" says Marsha Hudnall, MS, RD, program director of Green Mountain at Fox Run, a woman's retreat for healthy living in Ludlow, Vt.

Remember the connection between thoughts, emotions, and behaviors, says Hudnall. "The first feeds the second; the second, the third," she says. "If our thinking is awry, so go our emotions, and our behaviors reflect how we're feeling."

"Be alert to these common thinking errors," says Hudnall:

All-or-nothing thinking – the tendency to go to extremes and judge yourself and your body as extremely good or extremely bad. Change this thinking by recognizing that few things are truly black and white. "Should" statements – trying to motivate yourself with "shoulds", including comparing yourself to "perfect" images on television, the movies, or magazines.

Magnification/minimization – over-focusing on things you dislike about yourself while minimizing your positive attributes. Thank someone who compliments you and skip the "but."

Scapegoating – assuming that a physical characteristic you dislike about yourself is responsible for certain difficulties you encounter. Making assumptions and taking things personally can be a big mistake; fat prejudice does exist, but it's probably not responsible for all your troubles.

Emotional reasoning – thinking something must be true, if you feel or believe it. Identify what you are feeling, and remind yourself that it's just a thought -- which doesn't necessarily make it true.

"Living like a thin person also means thinking about food and eating in a different way," says Hudnall. "Are you hungry or satisfied? Do you like a particular food or not?" she asks. Those questions often don't come into play with people who struggle with food issues.

"Be in the moment," Hudnall advises. "Think about whether you're really hungry. Think about the taste of what you're eating. Don't be caught up in preconceived ideas of what you should or should not do."

That means you don't necessarily have to forgo ice cream. But really pay attention to what you're eating. If you do, one scoop should satisfy you as much as an entire pint. "It's really about being mindful," says Hudnall.

Ellen Astrachan-Fletcher, PhD, professor of clinical psychology and founder/director of the Eating Disorders Clinic at the University of Illinois Medical Center, wants people to focus not so much on being thin, but on being healthy and fit.

"My main goal is to help people think about food in terms of nutrition and energy – the reasons we need food in our lives," she says.

Focus on Health and Fitness

"People with weight issues too often see food as more meaningful than it really is," Astrachan-Fletcher says. "Food is not comfort; it's not a method of coping. Changing how you think about food and its role in your life will help you think, and live, like a healthy person."

A healthy person, for example, doesn't use food as a substitute for personal relationships. "If you're feeling lonely," says Astrachan-Fletcher, "explore social options and make new friends."

"A healthy person also incorporates exercise into his or her life," Astrachan-Fletcher adds. "Exercise is not only part of a successful weight loss or weight management program, but it also helps you alleviate, or even avoid, depression, stress, and anxiety."

Develop Your Skills

"To reach your weight loss goal (or any goal, for that matter), you must develop a set of skills that will help you become successful," says Howard Rankin, PhD, psychologist for the international support group TOPS (Taking Off Pounds Sensibly), and author of *The TOPS Way to Weight Loss: Beyond Calories and Exercise.*

Some of the skills that will help you live your way to a thinner, healthier body is:

- ✓ **Patience:** Take things one step at a time. Give up one of your "downfall" foods at a time, for example, not all of them at once.

- ✓ **Visualization:** Think about a specific situation you're going to encounter and how you will deal with it. "See" yourself going out to dinner and eating a healthy meal.

- ✓ **Accountability:** Rely on a support group, friends, or even a therapist to whom you have to report.

- ✓ **Self-Control.** Realize that every time you resist successfully, you're developing self-control. Congratulate yourself each time you do this.

- ✓ **Goal Setting:** Think in terms of small goals. You don't need to lose 60 pounds; all you need to lose is one pound next week. Each small goal you achieve will reinforce your motivation and set you up for success.

✓ **Journaling:** Keep a written account of your actions, your thoughts, and your feelings, as well as what you eat. This not only increases your self-awareness, but also helps you let out feelings you may try to "stuff" back in with food.

✓ **Assertiveness**: Learn to say no. Ask yourself, "Is this going to get me closer to my goal or further away?"

Remember the Rest of You

Finally, remember that you are more than someone who is trying to lose weight. This is especially true if you're a woman.

"Women tie too much of their self-esteem on their body image, which is likely to be distorted in a negative way, and not enough on other factors of their life," says Salvatore Cullari, PhD, professor emeritus of psychology at Lebanon Valley College in Annville, Pa.

"The more 'possible selves' a woman has," says Cullari, "the less likely she is to be overwhelmed by body image issues, which can lead to self-consciousness, depression, vulnerability, and crash dieting."

"Avoid even thinking about the aspect of yourself that makes you feel inferior, like your body, and focus on another aspect of your life in which you are very successful," says Cullari. "For example, you may be a businessperson, a mother, a wife, a doctor, a gardener, a skier, etc. Allow yourself to concentrate on those other aspects of your life where you feel more satisfied."

Weight Loss

Everybody who has ever eaten junk food knows that it leaves the body with further cravings for food and it doesn't really give you much energy. Junk food certainly causes weight problems and because of some of the contents of junk food, we destroy good cells and cause disease such as cardiovascular disease. If we go on very low calorie diets, which are sometimes recommended, we feel like we are starving, we crave real food, we end up with various diseases, and we generally have no energy.

Proponents of various weight loss diets supplement these depressive aspects of dieting with a variety of medications that speed up the nervous system, such that one generally forgets about being hungry. Unfortunately, the body does not.

So if we eat a lot of junk food we end up with storing the excess food, particularly the fat that we cannot use and it usually ends up in the wrong places. Whereas, if we eat food that is more nutritious we stop craving the junk food. This is because we maintain an ideal weight there is both physical and mental satisfaction, and we have a high level of energy when the proper food is eaten.

Healthy Eating

When we talk about proper food we're breaking that down into the basic food groups of:

- Fruits and vegetables
- Protein, including legumes
- Meat, fish,
- Grains,
- Beans
- Nuts
- Complex carbohydrates
- Whole grains
- Essential fats, which can come from seeds nuts and certain vegetables.

If we include in our diet a sufficient amount of highly nutritious essential food nutrients we do not crave food, we do not starve, and we can lose weight. One has to look at weight loss as not being on a diet, but rather being on a proper eating program. One wants to be eating as many natural foods as possible not achieving this goal with drugs or stimulants.

Healthy Weight Loss

A proper weight loss program means not starving but eating when you need to. It also means not burdening one's self with counting calories weighing food, or other obsessive compulsive behaviors, which many diets insist upon to make the individual cognizant of their food intake but rather to ingrain in one's self the knowledge of proper food intake.

If we eat a proper diet, we will burn fat naturally, and lose the excess fat, while at the same time adding appropriate amounts of muscle mass. When one is interested in developing muscle mass as most athletes are, it is vitally important that the proper foods are eaten so that the bulk, which is developed, is not useless bulk but the proper nutrients to develop muscles in an appropriate way. It is important that one looks at weight loss and weight maintenance as a lifetime goal, and not merely as a short-term venture to get into that favorite swimsuit.

Many studies have shown that binge eating and binge dieting is not only relatively unsuccessful on the long term, but also can be very detrimental to cardiovascular health. Being fat is not just about looking fat and being uncomfortable in a swimsuit. It is about quality of life because being overweight increases the risk of heart disease, cancer, stroke, high blood pressure, type-two diabetes, gall bladder disease and arthritis.

Antioxidants and Free Radicals

Antioxidants are chemicals that come from plants that neutralize free radicals. They are generally classified as phytochemicals. Humans have lost the ability to manufacture most antioxidants, so we must eat them in our diets.

Plants of course have the ability to produce these antioxidants, which protect them from the free radicals that are caused by sunlight. So if we eat the plants that have the antioxidants, we also protect ourselves against the free radicals.

Free radicals can be considered toxin that results from bringing the food that we need for energy. Burning food is like burning gasoline in a car it produces toxins. Inside us, the engine that burns the food is the mitochondria.

When the food is burned free radicals are produced they are missing an electron. These missing electrons search for another electron to flow its compliment. Usually it steals this missing electron from healthy cells. When a cells ability to make energy has gone down, because of missing electrons the cell gets sick if enough cells get sick it can cause us to lose energy develop various diseases, gain weight, show signs of aging, and develop various other aspects of degenerative diseases.

There are thousands of antioxidants that work to protect us from the plant world. Vitamin C, Vitamin E and Beta Carotene are the most well known.

There are many others and there is evidence that we need all of them working in synergy to get the most effective use out of these antioxidants.

Other studies have shown that we need these antioxidants to prevent the aging of not only the cells but of the entire body. Similarly, if the body is not stressed by too many calories, too many toxins, and too much of the wrong food, it will produce less free radicals and the degradation products of those free radicals.

Therefore, it will keep one's weight down which decreases the overall risk of developing heart disease etc. This puts the body at risk but will also decrease the degradation of the body itself.

Studies have shown that a diet that is high in vegetables and fruit will lead to a reduced risk of coronary heart disease, stroke, and various cancers. It appears that the high levels of natural anti oxidants (Carotenoids, Tocopherols (Vitamin E) and Ascorbic acid (Vitamin C) appear to be responsible for these reductions in risk.

The studies do not collaborate that taking these as supplements decreases cardiovascular disease in those that already have it. (Reference: Morris DL, Kripchevesky sb, Davis ce.)

According to the Lipid Research Clinics Coronary Primary Prevention Trial and a follow up study, JAMA, 1994, antioxidants appear to have multiple and synergistic interactions, and also exhibit properties of showing compartmentalization and tissue specificity. Because of this, it appears desirable to use either a plentiful diet of mixed vegetables and fruits, or to supplement with products that simulate combinations of chemo protective substances, i.e., the antioxidants.

Some of the positive nutrients are in fruits and vegetables.

Fruits

- ✓ Apples – are a good source of Boron and Vitamin C Boron has been shown to increase mental alertness, and boost estrogen in postmenopausal women. It is also known to reduce cholesterol, and contains significant Anti oxidants.

- ✓ **Cherries** – are a rich source of calcium, vitamin C, and anthocyanins. These can be very beneficial for osteoarthritis prevention.

✓ **Cranberries** – have a natural anti–bacterial and anti–viral activity particularly within the bladder.

✓ **Dates** – are high in an aspirin–like substance and boron. They also have a laxative effect.

✓ **Oranges** – contain many antioxidants including betacarotene, terpenes, flavonoids, and vitamin C.

✓ **Papaya** – is a rich source of potassium and vitamin A. It is well known to help with digestion.

✓ **Peaches** – are a good source of boron and contain vitamin C and betacarotene.

✓ **Pineapples** – are high in manganese and bromelain. Bromelain suppresses inflammation and aids in digestion. There is some evidence that it helps dissolve blood clots and prevents osteoporosis.

✓ **Prunes** – are well known as a laxative because of the high fiber content. The sweetness of prunes comes from sorbitol.

Selected Vegetables

✓ **Beets** – are high in folic acid and contain calcium, iron, and potassium.

✓ **Broccoli** – contains many of the antioxidants such as beta carotene, vitamin C and Indoles. It is cardio-protective and helps maintain lower cholesterol levels. There is a lot of calcium in broccoli and there is also a high level of Chromium.

✓ **Cabbage** – contain a number of antioxidants. These have been linked to various anti cancer, anti ulcer, and anti bacterial functions.

✓ **Carrots** – are an excellent source of beta carotene and other antioxidants. It has been linked to proper eye health for many centuries.

✓ **Kale** – is another source of antioxidants.

✓ **Parsley** – has a high level of antioxidants, such as monoterpenes, phthalides, and polyacetylenes. Parsley is also known to have diuretic activity, and to decrease blood clotting. There is a significant amount of folic acid in parsley.

✓ **Spinach** – has high antioxidants and significant amounts of fiber.

✓ **Tomato** – principal antioxidants are the lycopenes.

Fiber Sources

✓ **Cellulose** – Cellulose is a non-digestible carbohydrate found in the outer layer of fruits, vegetables and other plants. Cellulose is good at producing bulk in the gastrointestinal tract. Glucomannan is a fiber from a tuber plant called Amorphophallis. It normalizes blood sugar and helps curb appetite.

✓ **Pectins** – are fibers that come from the skin of apples and citrus fruits. It is known to assist in lowering cholesterol and removing various toxins from the body.

Weight Loss Complex

Dietary fiber complex-one wants a balance of insoluble and soluble fibers that help regularity in the G.I. tract, which cleanses and eliminates toxic waste.

Apple pectin, plant cellulose, complex carbohydrates, carrageenan (soluble fiber from green algae), locust, bean gum are good souces. Garcinia cambogia, a malabar tamarind fruit from Asia, suppresses appetite, enhances energy and increases fat burning.

Hawthorne Berries (circulation)

Chromium Stable (trivalent) assures mature absorption of carbohydrates and is an important cofactor for insulin function. This mineral is absent from many of our foods. Lecithin is important for normal fat metabolism. It helps to improve the digestion of fats, regulates storage of fats by helping to dissolve them and carry them through the blood stream.

Enzymes

Bromelain, papain, and protease help break down the proteins to amino acids for easy absorption.

Fibrinogen

Fibrinogen is the precursor of fibrin, a protein that plays a major role in the ability of blood to clot.

Although the exact relationship with coronary artery disease is not known exactly, we do know that fibrinogen interferes in some way with blood flow, which can contribute to intermittent muscle pain during exercise, high blood pressure, strokes and possibly atrial fibrillation.

We know that high blood sugar, very high cholesterol levels, exogenous estrogen, smoking, obesity, and stress will all increase fibrinogen levels in human beings.

We also know that to lower fibrinogen, exercise is the best agent. Fish oil supplements, garlic, vitamin E, a vegetarian diet and an occasional glass of wine will all lower fibrinogen levels.

Magnesium

Magnesium is an important mineral in the human body as it regulates how the body uses other nutrients, hormones, and vitamins. It is a co-factor for the proper utilization of various vitamins (vitamin B6, vitamin E), and is utilized in the process to break down, and adsorb protein.

It is found throughout the human body, and is vital to a majority of the biological processes we have. It is necessary for a healthy heart as it is involved in maintaining the integrity of blood vessels and relaxing smooth muscles (of which the heart is our largest). It also works in the process to maintain fluid and electrolyte balance and is critical in numerous enzyme reactions that control the metabolism of the body.

For example, magnesium is closely linked with calcium. Magnesium is needed to allow absorption of the calcium into the bones. Without the magnesium the calcium might be deposited in joints thereby causing arthritis.

Magnesium has been shown to increase the survival of patients who've had heart attacks. This apparently has to do with the fact that magnesium plays an important role in muscle contraction and cell integrity. Magnesium can allow oxygen to get to the heart muscle in times of need. A lack of magnesium can precipitate in abnormal heartbeat, called an arrhythmia.

Certain diseases are known to be associated with low magnesium – hypertension, kidney disease and diabetes are high on the list. It is also known that alcoholics have low magnesium, as do patients with chronic diarrhea. Increased stress can also lead to decreased magnesium.

Diets that are high in whole grains, fruits and vegetables tend to have sufficient magnesium for the bodies requirements. Food sources that are high in magnesium include whole grains like oats, brown rice, buckwheat, and millet. Legumes, such as lentils and beans, nuts, broccoli, bran, and chocolate are also high in magnesium.

Antioxidants

Antioxidants have various functions in the human body. They protect the human body by eliminating the adverse effects of oxygen. A simple example of this is the effect of lemon juice in keeping fruits fresh. Unstable oxygen molecules do damage when their electrons lose their partners.

If an oxygen molecule loses an electron it stabilizes itself by grabbing another molecule from any substance or tissue nearby to stabilize itself. Consequently it causes the other molecule to become unstable from the tissue that it has stolen it from. If a sufficient quantity of antioxidants isn't present, a chain reaction can take place with resultant damage to the tissue that has had molecules stolen from it.

This oxidation is what causes aging of cells and dysfunction of various body functions. These unstable oxygen molecules that steal from other tissues are called free radicals. The lemon juice and other antioxidants work by preventing the free radicals from doing further damage to other tissues.

They form a part of a well-balanced system that repairs oxidation damage and neutralizes the toxins that are there by produced. A normally healthy body is designed to keep free radicals in check, or directed to where they can be useful such as elimination of abnormal bacterial counts or viruses.

When oxidation goes out of control and free radicals are in very high quantities, damage such as heart disease can occur. Unfortunately, there are many free radicals in our environment such as found in cigarette smoke, pesticides, smog, and various preservatives, which are added to prepared foods.

Because it is very difficult to avoid some of these environmental free radicals it is vitally important that we eat plenty of fresh fruits and vegetables to fight the free radicals, and take various supplements that will also help in preventing disease and leading to a healthy heart.

Beta Carotene

Again eating lots of fruits and vegetables can provide this important ingredient on your diet, which is an antioxidant. Up to 25,000 international units a day is recommended as a supplement if sufficient dietary intake is not achieved. A number of studies have investigated beta carotene and heart disease. Some studies have shown impressive drops in all major coronary events and up to a 50% drop in other cardiovascular problems like stroke.

Unfortunately, the final word is not out on beta carotene as there are some current studies yet to be replicated that indicate that beta carotene is not as beneficial as previously felt.

The final word – Try to take sufficient quantities of spinach, carrots, yams and other vegetables and fruits that contain quantities of beta carotene but don't take too many supplements.

Glutathione

Glutathione is a protein made up of three amino acids – cysteine, glycine, and glutamic acid. It is found in the cells of almost all living organisms and is an important antioxidant. It catches free radicals before they start a chain reaction of destruction of normal cells.

It works in conjunction with vitamin E and selenium. In this latter combination it is very beneficial to the heart. There is some evidence that it is necessary to keep a low cholesterol level. Good sources of glutathione and its ingredient amino acids are found in yogurt, onions, garlic and wheat germ.

Ginkgo Biloba

Ginkgo Biloba and its active ingredient Ginkgo flavoglycoside is an active antioxidant. It is known to increase circulation to the heart and to the brain. It generally lowers bad (LDL) cholesterol and raises good (HDL) cholesterol.

Grape Seed Extract

Grape seeds, peanuts, cranberries, citrus peels, and lemon tree bark extracts are known to contain procyanidolic oligomers, a type of bioflavonoids. These bioflavonoids are strong antioxidants.

They are known to strengthen blood vessel walls and protect against adverse clotting. When combined with lecithin components it appears to be more effective in the human body.

Polyphenols

Polyphenols are organic compounds that act as potent antioxidants. They're particularly effective against fats in the body raise the good HDL and lower the bad LDL cholesterol. They also lower triglyceride levels that are known to have an effect on clotting of red blood cells. Polyphenols can be found in green tea. Caution needs to be raised when a patient has a certain cardiac condition because of the stimulant effect of green tea.

As mentioned in the beginning, antioxidants have a great protective effect against heart disease. They are health-promoting factors necessary for a healthy heart. Fresh fruits and vegetables are the best source of antioxidants including cauliflower, cabbage, broccoli, spinach, green vegetables, and yellow vegetables, such as onions, garlic, carrots, and sweet potatoes. Most fruits, when eaten fresh, contain some vitamin C.

Vitamin C

Vitamin C has been shown in studies to be a protective factor against heart disease. In fact, Vitamin C is important for a wide range of bodily functions from the healing of wounds, to the adjunctive prevention of viral diseases, to the production of certain anti stress hormones. Vitamin C works directly and in conjunction with other vitamins and enzymes in preventing various aspects of disease that contribute to heart disease.

For example, Vitamin C acts with vitamin E in the prevention of oxidation of unsaturated fatty acids and LDL (bad cholesterol). Vitamin C acts as an anti-clotting agent, which prevents damage to the coronary arteries.

One study demonstrated that redevelopment of thromboses (clots) in post surgical bypass patients was less if they took one gram of Vitamin C daily. Vitamin C works against the LDL cholesterol that is oxidized within the body. Anyone who has eaten too much fresh fruit will know that vitamin C can also act as a laxative.

This laxative action speeds up the removal of bioacids from the bowel. Bioacids are excreted into the intestines being composed from cholesterol. If the body needs more cholesterol it will reabsorb some of the bioacids and reconstitute cholesterol.

Consequently, if you increase the bio acid production as vitamin C does, you will increase the excretion of cholesterol. Vitamin C like other vitamins helps raise the good HDL cholesterol.

Vitamin C has been shown to help in keeping blood pressure decreased. We all know that our blood pressure needs to be kept under control both the systolic (upper) and diastolic (lower) blood pressure.

The best source of vitamin C is fresh fruits, especially citrus fruits. Vitamin C can also be taken as a supplement with 500-milligram tablets being easily available in most drug stores. While the RDA's recommended dosage of vitamin C is 500 milligrams, to have a healthy heart at least 1,000 milligrams a day should be consumed. B vitamins need to be increased if you are taking higher doses of vitamin C because vitamin C can help wash out certain B vitamins.

Stress, viral illnesses, major lacerations and smoking all decrease the body's level of vitamin C and increase the need for added supplementation. Patients with heart attacks have been shown to have significantly lower levels of vitamin C, and following a heart attack it is prudent to add vitamin C to the regimen.

Vitamin E

Vitamin E is well known as a healthy heart vitamin. Epidemiological studies of various populations have shown that those with higher levels of vitamin E in their diet had lower rates of coronary heart disease.

Other studies have shown that many Americans have very low vitamin E intake, which is particularly correlated with those populations who have high heart related disease.

Various studies have shown that approximately a 40% lower risk of heart disease can be demonstrated in populations that take either dietary or supplemental vitamin E.

Studies have shown that vitamin E inhibits the release of various clotting agents in the blood stream that can cause deleterious clumping and the risk of stroke or heart attack.

This is also advantageous in decreasing the effects of decreased blood flow to the lower extremities (claudication). Studies have shown that taking vitamin E can decrease the pain of claudication. It increases the potential for oxygen to get to the heart.

Vitamin E is an antioxidant. It reduces the levels of oxidized fat in the blood stream. It is important that it works with glutathione that is necessary for a healthy layer of cells that line the heart blood vessels and lymph channels.

Vitamin E is a fat-soluble vitamin and is found in a variety of nuts and seeds, soybeans, dark green leafy vegetables and fruit. It comes as tocopherols in both alpha and beta forms. For a healthy heart, 400 to 800 IU is good and safe at these high doses.

The dry form is better absorbed and does not add any extra fat to the diet. It works in conjunction with vitamin C, the flavonoids and selenium in addition to other cofactors.

Potatoes

As you are well aware, having sufficient complex carbohydrates in the diet is very important. Furthermore, eliminating fat and calories are also important in weight loss. And for most other health related programs.

Why potatoes? Potatoes are a very rich source of complex carbohydrates and amino acids. They are a good source of vitamins, fibers, and minerals. They're even an excellent source of protein with two grams of protein for every hundred grams of potato. This approaches the benefit of an egg in as far as essential amino acids are concerned. Two hundred and fifty grams of potatoes provide 25% to 35% of all the essential acids that are needed in a day.

But doctor, aren't potatoes fattening? If you were to ask your doctor this question, you would learn that potatoes are not fattening. A hundred grams of potatoes is only 85 calories. This is very low. Of course, this means that the potato had to be baked, boiled, or steamed – not fried, sautéed or smothered in cream sauce. That's when potatoes start costing lots of calories and fat.

Vitamins

There are a number of vitamins that are easily assimilated from the potato. A hundred grams of potato contains approximately forty milligrams of vitamin C. Baked potatoes preserve more of the vitamin C, in fact 250 grams of baked potatoes can actually provide the entire daily requirement of vitamin C.

Depending on the resource you search, one finds there are over forty–five different types of potatoes, each one having a slightly different flavor. Consequently, one could spend many an interesting meal trying various kinds and flavors of potatoes, and allowing oneself good complex carbohydrates, low calories, good fiber source and good vitamins.

Thallotherapy (Thalassotherapy) and Losing Weight

Thalassotherapy or Thallotherapy is one of those untested old time methods that has been used for many years as a treatment for excess weight in general, and excess weight in certain areas of the body. Generally, at least an hour and a half to two hours a day are spent in seawater, or its products. This is accomplished either as soaks, algae paste/marine mud applications, or warmed showers or massages with sea products.

This technique presumably allows for a lymphatic drainage and loss of excess fluids from the body, which is why they require one to drink water on a regular basis. Theoretically, the loss of fluids from the body is attached to toxins, which are eliminated through the use of the seawater.

It is said that in Thallotherapy, loss of volume of heavy legs and a general feeling of lightness is "almost automatic". Often, this technique is merely a reshaping of an extremity, and not necessarily a total loss of weight.

Modern thalotherapy for weight loss also includes beautification techniques and other aesthetic therapies Movement therapy and reeducation in water, and various other activities swimming in seawater are utilized to decrease body weight and increase muscle activity and certainly do no harm.

Most of these programs state that they can help somebody lose about five pounds in a two-week period. Obviously, as part of their programs, they put patients on very stringent diets.

Granted having food at Saint-Malo, Quibron, and Carnac with well-known chefs is a nice way of having dietetic weight reducing food. Some of the resorts will have a private dietitian who will specifically assist the patient in problem areas.

My experience in both English and French facilities is that often times the portions are very small and the food is very simple.

- ☑ It is true that generally one can lose some weight with this particular method of weight loss.
- ☑ It is accepted that to lose more than just a few pounds a minimum of two weeks is necessary.
- ☑ It is accepted that a change in lifestyle and particularly in dietary lifestyle is necessary to accomplish a true change in long-term weight loss.

Traditional Thalotherapy Treatment For Heavy Limbs.

A number of specific treatments are utilized for individuals with "thunder thighs", "elephant limbs" – or as more politely put by the French – "jambes lourdes". These include seawater exercises, water jets in the pool, sea water showers, alternating hot and cold water for the feet, walking in cold seawater and doing various exercises in the sea water. Lymphatic drainage, physical therapy, pressure therapy with glass bottle pressure on the limbs mechanically, and circulation treatments are all used.

Often these centers will also have various aqua gym exercises for the lower extremities and then claim within a week they can reshape large thighs.

Some of the centers will utilize other exercise programs circulatory massage, gym classes, saunas and steam room treatments.

Thalotherapy and Anti-Stress Treatment.

Classic thalotherapy has been redefined again for the treatment of stress. Here, one sees quite a few different showers that are used with seawater, with bubbling water, and combined with massages. There are also rest periods that are utilized in solariums and certain rooms that have deionized air in them so that one breathes in this deionized air for treatment of stress.

Sophrology, a technique consisting of a set of physical and mental exercises for reducing stress, and promoting well-being is often included in most of the thalo therapy treatment programs. Some resorts advertise sun and sea as a means of anti-stress, music in the swimming pool, facial therapy, acupuncture, and energetic re-equilibration.

A center in France advertises a private psychotherapist for weeklong participants of their stress program. Post-natal thalotherapy is the latest vogue in thalotherapy cure, which treats the mother after she has had a baby. These are specific programs that address the fatigue and emotions that surround having recently had a baby, and now having to deal with all the extra work and weight. Most traditional halo therapy centers will offer a postnatal program, and now are also adding massage courses for the mothers on how to massage their babies.

Another Medical Weight Loss Program

The Institute of Nutrition and Corporal Esthetics has implemented this new program for medically controlling weight loss and giving the parameters for continued weight control following the program.

This is both a physical and psychological approach to weight loss, which aims for a lasting weight loss cure. It utilizes all forms of thalotherapy, body wraps, dietary changes and mild exercise.

There is a team of specialists including a physician, dietitian, sophrologist, kinestheo therapist in addition to the thalotherapy specific treatment such as hydro massages, jet showers, aqua gym there are aesthetic treatments such as massage, lymphatic drainage, ultra sound, frigid therapy, etc.

The dietary changes are such that although the food has virtually no fat and very little calories, sous chefs have developed menus and recipes so that subtle flavors abound and the gourmet food is delicious. Being hungry is not part of this program.

Exercising in Deep Water

The rationale for utilizing exercise in deep water goes way back to the Greeks. If you could see what type of therapeutic spas that they used, you would see them exercising paraplegics, arthritics and others needing treatment in deep pools.

They also believed that the various properties of the specific waters had an influence on the treatment. This latter belief has been carried forth in many cultures and is the basis for many of the spas around the world that contain "curative waters".

Now in the 21st century, on a more physiological basis, we have shown that exercise in deep water can play an important role in various kinds of rehabilitation. The versatility of the movements and the physical properties of the water itself, allow deep-water exercise programs to be developed in a variety of settings for a number of conditions at all ages. Although I learned to swim at a very early age, in water therapeutic programs, one does not even need to know how to swim.

There are many therapeutic benefits to exercising in water, even shallow water. The most obvious of which is that there is no impact or contact with solid surfaces. The movement of the body part stops when the end of the range of motion is reached, or upon volition of the patient. Exercise in the pool can have zero impact, as is the case in deep water and minimal contact in shallow water exercises.

Gravity works in opposition to buoyancy in water, so that its effect is hardly noticed. This is in contradiction to any exercise that is done out of the water where the compressive effect is evident in the joints of the spine and lower extremities.

Therefore during deep-water exercise, buoyancy supports the body and protects the weight bearing joints. The only other place that this can be done is in outer space where one is out of the gravitational pull of the earth. Unfortunately, at this point in the new millennium, it is not practical to send patients to outer space for rehabilitation.

Because the amount of loading experienced by the body is a function of immersion in the water, deep-water exercise creates no pain from impact forces and compliance with exercises is better.

Just having an individual in the water can create a treatment in itself. In deep water, the patient's spine experiences mild traction. The compressive force of gravity is counteracted by the buoyant effect of water.

This effect can be increased by the use of weights on the hips or ankles, along with a flotation device at chest level. During this mild traction, intradiscal pressure decreases, for a minimal size increases, and there may also be some gapping of the facet joints. This is most likely the reason that patients with low back pain can exercise with considerably less discomfort in water than on land.

We know that all body parts from the neck down are submerged under water, and there is a greater surface area of resistance during exercise. Movements in water use all the major muscle groups, working the prime movers and the antagonist's muscles alternatively. This is called reciprocal strengthening. It is the basis for many physical therapeutic techniques (Rood, Proprioceptive Neuromuscular Facilitation-PNF, etc).

It provides muscular balance through the full range of motion and helps to reveal any imbalances that might exist. Because the hydrostatic pressure that acts on the submerged parts is equal and constant, imbalances may be identified and corrected.

Unfortunately, specific literature documenting increases in muscular strength and endurance with deep-water exercise is sparse. There are studies that show that water running is effective in maintaining leg strength in runners.

Based upon my own clinical observations, deep-water exercise is especially beneficial for sedentary patients, who want to maintain or increase their general strength while recovering from injuries or elective surgeries.

For patients who have had specific lung problems or in other ways need to strengthen the muscles of respiration, the hydrostatic pressure of the water itself provides a mild resistance to chest expansion in deep water. The intercostals and diaphragm must work harder, thereby strengthening those muscles.

The old rules of physics apply to water exercises. The resistance experienced by the body part in a certain exercise, depends upon the force exerted in the water. Resistance increases in response to the force exerted and stops immediately when the force is removed. It allows maximum control so that the patient can exercise in a pain-free or minimal pain range.

Another advantage of water exercise is that there is no eccentric muscle activity. This means that the resistance of the water slows the movement of an extremity, so that the patient's muscles are not required to do so. An example, is water running where only one half to one third the speed is required to obtain the same metabolic intensity as seen on land.

Here, micro-trauma to bones and muscles that can occur during the eccentric component of land-based exercise is absent. When you have an athlete who has injured him/herself, water exercise can be an important aspect of their treatment, as they do not perceive that they have to "rest" anything. At the same time, by not stressing the injured tissue, they are actually resting it while still exercising in the water.

We all know that maintaining aerobic conditioning is important. During an injury, post surgically, or with an elderly individual, this is often a real challenge in a rehabilitation program. Water exercises can be used to maintain the aerobic aspect of conditioning during the healing process without leading to more specific injuries in the damaged body part.

In the case of the elderly patient, although a lifetime of 'body damage' cannot be cured, water exercises can gently 'condition without damage'. Water exercises can also be used as a progression to more difficult levels of exercise.

Considering again the laws of physics, one must also consider what happens while you have a patient in the watery environment. The metabolic responses observed during some exercises in water are different from the same activity on land.

For example, during deep water running VO2max (maximum oxygen uptake), and maximal heart rate are seen to be lower than that on a treadmill exercise. This allows exercise at lower heart rates. The ambient temperature of the water can have an influence on the level of exercise and the calories expended.

Any swimmer knows that if you jump into a cold lake you will quickly lose body heat. Exercise vigorously in that cold environment and you will be able to feel warmer. It takes more energy to feel comfortable than being in bath water.

If you have a patient who is already having to direct a great deal of the body energy to the healing process, the last thing you want to do is to use up some of that precious energy in just warming the body temperature to a comfortable level to do exercise.

In the extreme, if the water is too cold for the recovering patient, a mild form of hypothermia (the lowering of the body temperature similar to what happens if you fall into the ocean in the winter) can occur, even in water that feels ok to the average person. Similarly, if the water is too warm, the body will expend valuable energy in trying to keep the body temperature stable and not overheat.

Ideally in most situations, one wants the temperature of the water for exercise to be slightly cool in the vicinity of 28–30 degrees centigrade (82–86 degrees Fahrenheit) for aerobic activities to prevent the body from storing heat during the exercise.

One must also consider the outside ambient temperature. If the air temperature is a sunny 85 degrees, a cooler water temperature is indicated. If it is a cloudy 55 degrees air temperature, a slightly warmer water temperature is okay.

Exercise can be done in the fresh air in certain parts of the world all year long, and obviously needs to be put inside at various times of the year in other climes. Exposure to sun, which we will discuss in detail in other areas of the book, should be kept to a minimum due to not only the damaging effects of UV light, but also the 'energy draining effect' it has on a patient who is trying to recover from some other condition.

One should also consider the chemicals added to the water being exercised in. Some individuals are allergic to certain pool chemicals such as chlorine, bromine, algaecides, etc. Others have skin reactions to some of the pool clarifiers.

If exercising in fresh water (lakes, rivers, ocean), consider the bacteriologic and arthropod population that may affect the individual. I well remember a crystal clear lake near where I was practicing in Seattle, Washington that gave at least 4 individuals a day (whom I saw in my practice) schistosomiasis, more commonly known as swimmer's itch.

There is another well-known lake in Seattle, WA that is an *in place* to live around. Many people wind surf on it, swim in it, and bask by its shores. By midsummer, it grows a very heavy population of algae that can cause an itchy rash. This algae gets so thick at times that people have actually been known to have gotten tangled in it and nearly drowned.

Exercising at the ocean beach has another whole set of potential complications. Undertows and riptides can be potentially fatal to the weaker swimmer. Stepping on a sea urchin spine, being bitten by a crab, or getting a laceration from a piece of glass on the beach must all be prepared for. It is one thing to get conditioning for a patient and totally another if they are attacked by jellyfish in the process!

On the other hand, exercise at the beach can be not only effective, but also diverting for the patient. Seeing the scenery at the beach can take their mind off the whole rehabilitation process. The fresh air is certainly also better than the stale air of an institution.

At a beach where there is plenty of wave action, just standing and maintaining one's balance will provide a good workout for the muscles of the lower extremity. When those muscles are strong enough, move to increasingly deeper water to increase the resistance. The added resistance of the wave action at a beach can augment some upper extremity and core exercises.

When exercises are performed in deep water, the body should be held vertically with the abdominal and gluteal muscles contracted. Considering the physics of being in the water again, one sees that the center of gravity in deep water shifts to the chest from where it is on land, which is around the symphysis pubis (pelvis).

This creates a turning or buoying effect on the body, which must be counteracted by muscular activity. This is good for the patient who is stable enough. Sometimes it is better to provide a belt or buoyancy vest to the patient so that they can maintain the correct vertical position, which is the water line at shoulder level and the head comfortably out of the water.

The specific exercises that are beneficial to the specific individual should be worked out with a physical therapist that is familiar with water exercises.

There are many different techniques that have been developed. Some therapists apply land-based programs to the water: PNF in the water, water Yoga, water jogging, etc.

Others have developed a variety of specific water exercises. All can have beneficial effects and should maintain or enhance muscular strength and endurance and general level of fitness. They must all address correct body alignment so that no damage is done to the body.

Examples of the type of exercises that are specific for the water include those in the paragraph below. These types of exercises are self-explanatory from the name, but performing them correctly so that the maximum benefit is gained for the effort expended requires the advice of a Physical Therapist.

Deep water exercises for the lower body could include jogging, walking, bicycling, stride jumping, lunges, abdominal knee lifts, flutter kicking, hip abduction, flexion & extension, gluteal squeezing, etc. Exercises for the upper extremities could include the breaststroke, crawl, bent & straight-arm pulls, shoulder circles, shoulder and elbow presses, pull ups with the pool steps, side pushups, etc.

All in all, water exercise, and deep-water exercise in particular can play an important role in not only routine fitness, but also an especially important method of rehabilitating various parts of the body after injury or long-term disabilities.

Your Metabolic Rate

We all want to and try to control our metabolic rate in the hopes of getting the perfect body weight. What is it and what is it not? Metabolism is the body's systems that use or convert energy. This includes digestion, muscle building, and breathing. It also, of course, includes the storage of fat circulation of the blood and any other activity that converts energy into an activity you need to live.

There are 2 different metabolic processes that occur in your body.

1. Anabolic reactions, which involves building cellular structures and storing of energy.

2. Catabolic reactions, which involves breaking down molecules for energy.

Your metabolic rate is the speed of your metabolism, or the rate at which you burn calories. The metabolic rate at which you burn calories while your body is at rest is otherwise known as your basal metabolic rate.

In general, the more muscle and less fat you have, the higher or faster your metabolic rate. Your metabolic rate is strongly influenced by your body composition. A high protein diet particularly high plant-based protein diet requires more energy to process. This means that your metabolic rate increases when your body has to digest high fiber high protein plant-based foods. Men tend to have higher metabolic rates than women.

Your metabolic rate is determined by a number of factors, genetics being one of the important ones. Diet and exercise can also play an important role, and unfortunately as we grow older our metabolic rate tends to slow down. Beginning in your 20s, your metabolic rate begins to decline at approximately 2% every 10 years

Your thyroid gland is the main regulator of metabolism. The thyroid hormones determine how fast or slow you burn calories, store fat and integrate with how certain other hormones work. Malfunction of the thyroid gland can lead to various conditions including weight loss and weight gain, but not in a healthy manner.

It was a fad in the 50s and 60s for physicians to give overweight patients extra thyroid hormone to assist them in losing weight. It was quickly found that this was an undesirable practice, and it was found that if one controlled the thyroid to its ideal function, that a person could lose or gain weight in a much more healthy manner.

Drastically limiting calories does not assist you in raising your metabolic rate as a means of losing weight. Studies have shown that people eating less than 1200 calories per day are likely to end up with a slower metabolic rate and consequently do not lose the weight they expected. One's body is basically going in to slow down mode to potentially survive the presumed famine. In contradiction to starving, eating like a chicken (small but frequent meal, which helps boost calorie burn) is a good way to actually burn calories and increase the metabolic rate.

Stimulants, in the form of diet, and energy drinks and diet pills, are very popular in today's marketplace. These include power drinks, boost drinks, and of course the main ingredient caffeine. They will actually boost your metabolism by a few percent for a very short time.

Some spicy foods can actually also raise your metabolic rate. This will not necessarily help you lose lots of weight, but adding hot peppers (capsaicin) will produce thermo genesis (producing heat), which will burn a few calories.

If you live in a cold climate, your metabolism is forced to speed up to keep your body warm. And in hot weather your metabolism has to speedup to keep you cool. In general, it is the hot tropical climate that generally increases your metabolic rate anywhere from 5-20%. Unfortunately, when you live in a hot tropical climate, the body generally wants to slow down its activity to cool off.

You actually burn more calories just maintaining your body's vital processes than you do through physical exertion. 65-70% of the calories you burn in a day are burned by your metabolism in maintaining your body is vital processes. Physical exercise adds another 30% of daily calorie burn and it is the best way to boost your metabolic rate.

CHAPTER 17

HUMAN PERFORMANCE

AFFECTED BY DEHYDRATION

It is vitally important that you drink fluids and keep yourself hydrated. In many jobs and personal situations, it is required that people work at a specific pace to complete the tasks assigned. This requires peak performance mentally, physiologically, and physically.

The human body depends on numerous heat sensitive enzymatic and chemical reactions to function properly. To do this, the body must maintain the body's fluid balance at adequate levels. Although many people are truly athletes physically and mentally in their private lives, many do not adhere to the same precepts as professional athletes do in maintaining appropriate hydration. There is a physiological fact that the rate of voluntary fluid intake, after fluid depletion, is slow in man as compared with most other mammals.

Using the fact that working in a hot environment dehydrates people and makes them less efficient, I performed a study. I hypothesized that if one forces people to consume fluids, it improves their performance.

To study this, I designed a prospective controlled intervention research project. To do this, a group of 256 Mexican factory workers were tested for various arms of the study.

A careful review of medical histories was carried out. Those with cardiac, renal, or endocrine problems or a history of adverse reactions to hot environments were eliminated from the study. All participants were given a mini-physical examination where general health, vital signs, urinalysis, blood sugar, range of motion, and grip strength were documented.

Of the original group, a subset was chosen that had similar baseline characteristics. Differences in age, body habitus, length of time on the job, etc were matched.

All participants had similar positions in a manufacturing plant working on an assembly line with moderate physical exertion (by ILO classification). All had the same amount of break time.

Of the 256 participants, 206 had similar calculated performance time, as measured by the number of pieces and procedures each was required to perform per hour. Ambient plant temperature ranged between 38–40 degrees C. during all aspects of the study.

The first arm of the study was to test baseline hydration and mechanical efficiency (HME) of the study group. Before work and at the end of the shift, they underwent the HME test: Body weight & temperature, skin turgor, mucous membrane hydration, mini step test (number of steps achieved over 3 minutes), and grip strength on a Jamar Grip Tester. The entire HME test took less than 5 minutes.

The group was then individually subjected to exercise during the day to produce profuse sweating (jogging in place, & sit-ups). HME testing was done before & after the exercise.

Next, 94 participants were chosen to be tested. These individuals were allowed to consume water as to their own liking. The HME test was performed at the end of the workday along with a self reported simple rating questionnaire of fatigue that was asked of the participants.

Subsequently, in the second arm of the study, the same group was required to consume a minimum of 4, and a maximum of 5 liters, of water that was provided to them, during their 9–hour workday. At the end of the day, they underwent the same HME test and fatigue questionnaire. Questionnaires from subjects' supervisors were evaluated for subjective performance change in the participants.

The results of this study were very telling for all people who want to stay healthy. Dehydration for this study was defined when a worker had a decrease of body hydration as measured by mucous membrane hydration, skin turgor, and body weight. The first group tested was found to be dehydrated after exercise in a hot environment by our above methodology. This coincided with an increase in body temperature.

Mechanical efficiency for this study was measured by changes in the step test and Jamar grip strength testing. Testing demonstrated that when dehydration amounted to 2%, that there was no significant decrease in the measured mechanical efficiency; but when the dehydration became 3%, that there was a statistically significant change (p>.01) in the mechanical efficiency.

94 individuals completed the study regarding the intake of water either ad lib (control) or being forced to consume a specific quantity of water (intervention).

In so much as the objective clinical measurements that were performed (HME) the intervention (forced to drink water) demonstrated better hydration, better mechanical efficiency, and lower average body temperature at the end of the workday in comparison to their prior results when they were allowed to drink ad lib.

Subjectively, the group consistently reported (questionnaire) less fatigue and a better ability to perform tasks during the test period when they were forced to drink fluids in comparison to the results when they were allowed to drink ad lib.

Supervisors reported that the group had better performance when forced to drink fluids than when they were their own control group and drank ad lib.

When allowed to drink as desired, the group drank significantly less water on average as compared to the interventional period.

It was concluded that heat induced dehydration can significantly affect mechanical efficiency and forced hydration can improve the performance in a group of otherwise healthy manufacturing plant workers, just think what it can do for you.

CHAPTER 18

DELICIOUS HEALTHY RECIPES

Beverages & Hors d'Ouevres

WEDDING PUNCH (COLD)

- 4 quarts pure cranberry juice (no added sugar or preservatives)
- 4 quarts sparkling water (no added sugar or preservatives)
- 2 quarts unsweetened apricot nectar
- 1/2 gallon of raspberry or strawberry Rice Dream (rice milk)

Mix together all the liquid ingredients and spoon the Rice Dream on the very top of the wedding punch. Keep everything cold. Set the punch bowl on ice while dishing up. Do not use ice in the punch, as it will dilute it. God Bless.

HEALTHY CHRISTMAS GLOG

- 2 quarts of natural cranberry juice (no sugar or sweetener)
- 10 cardamom seeds
- 5 sticks of cinnamon (pounded but not so the sticks peel off)
- 3 whole spice berries (pounded)
- 4 cups apple cider (no preservatives or sugar)
- 2 cups golden white raisins
- A couple of long strips from 2 small oranges
- A couple of long strips from 2 limes
- 2-1/2 cups slivered almonds

Put cinnamon sticks, cardamom seeds, 1/2 strips from oranges and limes into cheesecloth. Tie ends of cheesecloth together, toss it in with the other ingredients, heat and simmer.

Wash raisins and soak raisins in a little cranberry juice. Remove cheese bag. Serve the Glog hot in a large punch bowl. Garnish the rest of the orange/lime strips – put a lighted floating candle in the center of the Glog.

Have ready a bowl of drained raisins and a bowl of slivered almonds. Pour the Glog over almonds and raisins. Give each person a demi- tasse spoon. Merry Christmas.

PARTY PUNCH

- 2 packages frozen raspberries (unsweetened)
- 2–3 cups cherry juice (unsweetened no preservatives)
- 1 quart of sparkling water (no preservatives)

Mash raspberries and cherry juice, pour over ice cubes made out of cherry juice and add sparkling water last. Serve. Have a good party.

VEGETARIAN (MOCK) TUNA DIP

Tuna roll (there are several commercial brands like the one made by Worthingtons) this mock tuna tastes very much like real tuna.

- 1/2 roll defrosted
- 1–1/2 Tablespoon "Nayonaise" or homemade Soy mayonnaise
- 2 scant teaspoons dry soy milk
- 1 tablespoon soy sour cream
- 1/8 teaspoon garlic powder
- 1/4 teaspoon onion powder
- 1/4 cup finely cut seaweed (Nori or similar)
- Rice milk as needed

Put everything into a food processor but keep out 1/8 cup of seaweed for garnish. Chill. Just before serving, add 1/8-cup seaweed on top of dip.

CHILI RELLENOS (not fried, no dairy)

- Fresh green chilies (sweeter ones rather than the hot kind)
- Roast in oven or broil. Put them in a paper bag for 1/2 hour or more when cool
- Pick off skins and remove the seeds and veins
- Fill each rellenos with non-dairy white (soy) cheese and put peppers in rice milk

Dip the stuffed peppers in 1-1/2 cups of potato flour that has onion and garlic powder added. Grease non-stick cookie sheet. Place chili rellenos on cookie sheet and bake at 350 degrees. Turn once. Serve with a dab of non-dairy sour cream and a sprinkle of sweet paprika.

AFRICAN EGGPLANT DIP

- 1-1/2 lbs. eggplant (peeled)
- 1/8 cup white vinegar
- 1/2 cup small pitted green olives (not in oil)
- 3 ounces marinated artichoke hearts
- 1/8 cup of cashew butter
- 1/2 teaspoon cumin (ground)
- 2 tablespoons green onion tops

Steam peeled eggplant. Put everything in food processor. Blend well (until all is smooth as butter). Serve with baked corn chips. Garnish with a sprinkle of sweet paprika and finely chopped green onion tops.

AMERICAN SPINACH DIP I

- 1 package frozen spinach (thawed and drained)
- 1/4 cup green onion tops
- 1/2 cup soy mayonnaise
- 1/2 cup soy cream
- Garlic and onion powder to taste
- 1/2 teaspoon cardamom powder
- 1/2 teaspoon grated nutmeg

Puree everything together. Decorate dip with pimientos (can be purchased in glass jar). Drain well.

NON-DAIRY SPINACH DIP II

- 1 lb. fresh spinach (or if you must, 1 package frozen spinach thawed)
- 2 teaspoons ground mint
- 3 tablespoon non dairy sour cream
- 1/2 teaspoon grated nutmeg
- 1/4 teaspoon ground Cardamom
- garlic and onion powder to taste

Wash the spinach very well and dry well. Place in food processor with spices and non-dairy sour cream. Blend well. Chill. Serve with celery and carrot sticks. (Garnish spinach dip with cherry tomatoes and a sprig of mint).

MUSHROOM PATE
- 1 lb. fresh mushrooms
- 1/2 cup ground fresh parsley
- 1-1/2 tablespoons margarine mix
- 1-1/2 tablespoons Arrowroot dissolved
- 1/2 cup finely ground bread crumbs
- 1/8 teaspoon crumbled rosemary
- 1/8 teaspoon crumbled basil
- 2 bottoms of minced green onion tops

Garnish
- 1 tablespoon green onion tops
- 1-1/2 tablespoons of steamed sliced mushroom
- 1 teaspoon ground parsley

Sauté minced bottom of green onions in non-stick pan, mix with mushrooms. Mix in all ingredients and put into food processor. Spoon into a greased loaf pan. Bake in preheated oven, 375 degrees. Cover for about 1-1/2 hours. Check in 1 hour as it may be done. Chill well in refrigerator. Add garnish just before serving.

ORIENTAL SPICY RELISH DIP
- 1/2 teaspoon Cumin
- 1/2 teaspoon Ground cloves
- 1/2 teaspoon Cinnamon
- 1/4 teaspoon grated nutmeg
- 1 cup apple juice (fresh squeezed)
- Juice of 2 limes
- 2 teaspoons of arrowroot (stir well)
- 2 cups of pineapple fruit (fresh or unsweetened pineapple in its own juice)
- 1 teaspoon ginger
- 1/4 cup of dried onion flakes
- 1/4 teaspoon tamarack

Brown herbs in dry pan. Add other ingredients and bring to a boil. Simmer for 20 to 25 minutes. Refrigerate. Serve cold.

BAKED EGGPLANT SPEARS (with special sauce)

- 1-1/2 lb. oriental eggplants
- 3/4 cup potato flour
- 1/2 cup rice milk
- 1 teaspoon arrowroot powder dissolved
- 1/2 tsp. lemon thyme crumbled
- Garlic and onion powder (to taste)

Slightly oil the cookie tray. Slice the eggplant very thin, long thin slices. Dip the eggplant into rice milk that has the arrowroot powder well dissolved. In a plastic bag put garlic, onion powder, dill and lemon thyme mixed well with the potato flour.

Remove eggplant from rice milk. Place in a plastic bag and shake well. Remove eggplant from plastic bag and arrange on grease cookie sheet. Bake at 375 degrees for 20 to 25 minutes. Turn once; check that the eggplant is crisp (browned) on the outside and soft on the inside. Sprinkle a small brushing of paprika on eggplant and serve with dipping sauce in separate dishes. See dipping sauce recipe or chutney.

BERRY NON-DAIRY CHEESE DIP

- 1-1/2 cups fresh or frozen raspberries, (blackberries, strawberries or blueberries can be substituted), Do NOT use berries that are sugared or sweetened. Do use only one kind of berry.
- 1-1/2 teaspoons of dissolved arrowroot
- 8 ounces of white non dairy cheese
- 3/4 tablespoon of fresh lime juice
- 1 tablespoon of dry soy milk powder

Combine everything in a food processor until consistency of whipped cream. Garnish with berries (kind you used) and serve with dried apple chips or fruit spears like apple or pear.

SOY ONION DIP

- 1 cup firm tofu
- 1/8 cup rice vinegar
- 1/2 tablespoons dehydrated onions
- 1/2 teaspoon garlic paste
- 1 tsp. dried onion powder
- 1 tablespoon dry soy milk powder
- 2 tablespoons non-dairy soy sour cream
- 2 green onion stalks

Be sure powder is blended well. Combine all ingredients but the mild green onion tops. Blend to a creamy consistency. Garnish with finely chopped green onions on the top of the dip.

MIDDLE EASTERN DIP (HUMUS)

- 1 can of chickpeas (well drained)
- 1-1/2 teaspoon garlic paste
- 2 teaspoons each lime juice and lemon juice
- 2 teaspoons tahini
- 1 teaspoon (low sodium) tamari
- Sprig of parsley
- 1 teaspoon of lemon zest

Use food processor, mash well-drained chickpeas, tahini tamari and garlic. Increase or decrease garlic paste to taste. Add juice of the lime and lemon juice with a sprig of parsley and the fine grated peel of the lemon (lemon zest). Chill. Serve cold.

AFRICAN SNACK

- 2 cups whole wheat flour (pastry)
- 1 tsp. ground fresh ginger peeled
- 1/4 teaspoon ground cloves
- 1/2 teaspoon ground cinnamon
- 1/8 teaspoon ground fennel
- 1/8 teaspoon ground cardamom
- 1/8 teaspoon ground cumin
- 1/8 teaspoon nutmeg (ground)
- 1/8 teaspoon all spice ground
- 2 teaspoon pure maple syrup

Begin with 2/3-cup ice water in a non-stick pan, add brown herbs and stir. Put aside. Mix flour and water. Knead until there is thick dough. Add the herbs. Fold the dough over again. Cover the dough with a cloth.

Break off chunks of the dough and roll into strips. Cut a piece off long strip, using scissors. Bake on a non-stick greased baking cookie sheet at 350-degrees. Turn once. Serve as you would oriental mix.

GREEK DIP
- 2 large burpless cucumbers
- 1/2-cup soy sour cream (non-dairy)
- Garlic powder, onion powder to taste
- 1 teaspoon ground fresh mint
- 1/2 teaspoon dried mint

Peel and chop the cucumbers very fine. Mix all ingredients together. Chill well. Garnish with a few slices of cucumber to the top of the dip.

BABA GANOUI (Middle Eastern Dip)
- 1-1/2 teaspoon tahini
- 1 small fresh lime and 1 small lemon (juice from each)
- 1-1/2 teaspoon garlic paste (more or less to taste)
- 1 teaspoon (scant) liquid smoke
- 1 large eggplant or 1-1/4-lbs. Japanese eggplant

Peel eggplant. Cut off end of eggplant (if you are using Japanese eggplant). If using other large eggplant, bake eggplant in shell and scoop out insides. Peel and steam Japanese eggplant. Mash everything together with 1/2 teaspoon tahini. Garnish with a sprig of watercress. Chill. Serve cold.

HOT PEAR AND PEACH APPETIZER
- 1-lb. fresh pears and 1 lb. fresh peaches
- 1 tablespoon soy sour cream
- 1 tablespoon Non Dairy cheese
- 1 tablespoon finely grated ginger

Peel peaches, cut in half, remove core. Peel pears, cut in half, remove core. Broil until fruit is warm. Put a dab of sour cream and non-dairy cheese on each pear and peach. Return to the oven and heat until cheese starts to melt, sprinkle a touch of grated ginger on top of the fruit. Serve warm.

DOLMAS (Greek)

- 1 medium jar grapes leaves (well washed and soaked), remove as much salt as possible
- 1 small package of Sultanas
- 1-1/2-cups brown basmati rice
- 1 tablespoon dried onion
- 1 tablespoon dried parsley well crumbled
- 1-1/2 teaspoon dried mint leaves well crumbled
- 1 tsp. ground cardamom
- 1/4 cup white raisins
- 3-/4 tablespoon Japanese spiced vinegar
- 2 tablespoons pine nuts
- 1/2 cup orange juice (canned frozen concentrated)
- 1/4 cup lime juice (canned frozen concentrated)

Place grape leaves on pan with stems facing up toward you. Place mixture on each grape leaf. Fold grape leaves. Add orange juice and limejuice concentrate and spiced Japanese vinegar to the casserole dish.

Cover and bake until grape leaves are soft, for 1/2 hour to almost an hour. Be sure the dolma doesn't burn. Add a little hot water from time to time. Just brush a touch of olive oil on top of each dolma and add a couple of pine nuts on top.

MOCK TUNA SANDWICH

- Long thin whole wheat sour dough French bread (no preservatives or fat)
- Mock tuna frozen roll (made from tofu & gluten)
- 1 small jar artichoke hearts
- 1 large tomato thinly sliced
- 1 tablespoon treated sea weed finely cut
- 1/2 teaspoon dill weed finely crumbled

Slice fresh sourdough French bread the long way into 2 halves. Defrost the mock tuna - crumble it into small pieces, add seaweed that has been finely cut in thin strips. Drain artichoke hearts.

Sprinkle with dill weed; add thin slice tomato, more dill weed sprinkled on top of the tomatoes. Put the two halves of the loaf together. Press down, place loaf on a platter surrounded by sprigs of parsley. Enjoy.

PETITE SANDWICHES

- 1/2 cup plain non dairy cheese
- 1 teaspoon ground fresh dill
- 1/2 marinated artichoke hearts (cut very finely)
- 1/2 teaspoon lemon thyme crumbled well or 1/2 tsp fresh basil ground finely
- 1 teaspoon capers (drained)
- 1/2 tsp. Chives
- 1/2 tsp. parsley (ground)
- A few green olives (non oily)
- 1 tsp. green onion tops chopped very finely
- Alfalfa sprouts (very fresh)
- 1/2 small cucumber peeled and diced very finely
- Rye bread sliced very thin

Mix everything but capers, rye bread and alfalfa sprouts. Cut rye bread paper thin (health bread of rye flour). Spread with above mixture (there will be 3 layers). To each layer, add capers and a little alfalfa sprouts – 3 layers down. Add a toothpick with an olive in each sandwich.

STUFFED MUSHROOMS 1

- 2 lbs. large whole fresh mushrooms
- 1 tablespoon dried onion
- 1 teaspoon of fruit vinegar (ex. raspberry or strawberry)
- 2 teaspoons of olive oil
- Garlic powder to taste
- 2/3 to 1 cup dried (healthy) bread crumbs
- 12 tablespoons of white grated non dairy cheese
- 2-1/2 tablespoons parsley

Clean mushrooms. Cut off stems, (save stems). Place 1 teaspoon olive oil on a non-stick pan, brown non-dairy cheese and parsley. Lightly brush tops of mushrooms with a teaspoon of olive oil.

Mix ingredients and stuff the mushrooms. Bake at 350-degrees until mushrooms are tender. Top with remainder of ground parsley. Serve warm. If you have some cut pimiento you can place it on top as a garnish.

STUFFED MUSHROOMS-2

- 3/4 lb. mushrooms
- 1/2 to 3/4 cup healthy bread crumbs
- 3/4 tablespoon olive oil
- Garlic powder to taste
- 1/2 tsp. garlic paste
- 1 tablespoon ground parsley

Wash mushrooms, place in a wet cloth. Remove stems and use stems in soup, stir fries, etc.

Place mushrooms upside down (stem side up) in a greased non-stick dish. Brown bread crumbs that are very finely ground in a pan with garlic powder, garlic paste and ground parsley. Brown the mixture and stuff the mushrooms. Heat well at medium heat, serve hot.

ITALIAN ANTIPASTO

Antipasto is really like a platter of hors d'ouevres or a light supper.

- French bread (no preservatives, only flour, yeast and water). Serve in separate dishes.
- Marinate vegetables. Add cardamom powder. Let all marinate, chill and serve.
- Garbanzo beans: Use marinade, add Garam Masala and chill.
- Add beans, use marinade and add chili powder. Serve cold
- Marinate Mushrooms: sprinkle with garlic and onion powder.
- Red, green, yellow, purple peppers: Grill and remove skins. Marinate, chill and serve in long strips.
- Artichokes: Marinate: Add garlic and onion powder to taste. Serve cold (chill well).
- Sweet pickles/dill pickles (no alum preservative, no sugar)
- A dish of tofu wieners: cut in little rounds; marinate (a short time) stirring constantly. Add 1/2 - 1 teaspoon of smoke flavor. Heat. Keep

stirring on very low heat until wieners absorb all the marinade and smoke flavor. Present with strips of pimiento. Serve hot.

HOT PEARS WITH PINK BLANKET

- 6 fresh pears (slightly steamed)
- 1/4 teaspoon non-dairy white cheese per pierced pear
- 3/4 cup cherry cider or cherry juice (no preservatives, no added sugar or sweetener)
- 2 teaspoons dissolved arrowroot

Peel pears, steam slightly. Cut into 6 sections. Place 1/4-teaspoon non-dairy white cheese on each slice of pear. Add dissolved arrowroot to the cherry cider or cherry juice. Heat everything. Place pears on dish; pour "pink" cherry juice on top. Garnish with cherry.

FRUIT SMOOTHIES

Smoothies are a fast and healthy way to consume lots of nutrients in a pleasing tasty drink. It's an excellent morning starter. Fresh or frozen fruit only:

Fruit combo examples:

- Pineapple, pear, papaya, banana
- Fresh orange juice, banana, strawberries, tofu.
- Apple, banana, tofu, strawberries or raspberries
- Fresh orange juice, banana and fresh ginger
- Fresh grapes (seedless), mint and tofu
- Melon, fresh lime juice, mint

Hot fruit shakes: Apple juice, (fresh apples can be put through vegetable juicer), nutmeg, cinnamon and a touch of limejuice. Blend well in a juicer or blender.

With either the cold or hot versions, add 2 tablespoons of tofu or protein powder, a fiber mix, a few spinach leaves, and Stevia to taste (if it is not sweet enough). Be creative! It is amazing how you can really make a meal in a smoothie and get all your nutrients for a good morning starter or afternoon pick-me-up.

HEALTHY PARTY BEVERAGES

Fresh mixed vegetable juice can be taken every day. For example, juice from carrots, celery, parsley, cabbage and kale. If you do not have kale all the time, use broccoli, cabbage, dandelion greens, bok choy, etc. Some people enjoy beets in this veggie cocktail too. Remember you may use any greens you like but know that kale, cabbage, and some others can make your drink bitter.

Other standard combos:

- Add Spirulina or barley powder to increase the green effect
- Carrots and cucumber (more carrots if you like is sweeter)
- Carrots and cabbage
- Carrots and spinach
- Carrot, celery, cucumber, spinach, green pepper.

Mix and match for good health.

HERB TEA

There are many good herb teas on the market. Follow the directions on the box. Try fruit teas, experiment with your own blend. Do not use decaffeinated teas.

If possible make your herb tea a sun tea by putting tea or tea bags in a quart jar and standing the jar (with a tight lid) in the sun.

- Ginger is king when it comes to tea and so easy to make. Peel fresh ginger root, cut into small pieces put into boiling water in a pre-warmed teapot.
- Let it simmer.
- Strain and serve or add to other herbal teas.

Look at all the brands of boxed herb teas, read the labels and try them. Mix and match. Green tea, as we have discussed, has many benefits, but do remember it does have caffeine.

Sauces, Gravy, Chutney & Relish

REALLY GOOD TACO SAUCE

- 1 large can of tomatoes (no sugar or oils)
- 2 tablespoons dried onions
- 2 green peppers (chopped)
- 1 sweet red pepper (chopped)
- 2 tomatoes (peeled and chopped)
- 3 tablespoons parsley (ground)
- 3 bay leaves
- 1 teaspoon (each) oregano, basil, dill weed, chili powder, sage, sweet basil, cumin and paprika
- 1 tablespoon low sodium soy sauce
- 2 teaspoons lime juice.
- 1 cup chopped Seitan

Heat herbs in dry non-stick pain. Add 1/2 cup chopped seitan to 1/2 teaspoon garlic paste. Simmer all ingredients above, except the lime juice (you may have to add a few drops of water). Remove from stove and pour in limejuice.

TOMATO CREAM GRAVY

- 1 cup tomatoes
- 3/4 tablespoon dried onions
- 1/8 cup cashew pieces (raw)
- 1/8 cup brown rice cooked
- 2 pinches each: dill weed, parsley, oregano, thyme and mint
- 1/2 teaspoon garlic paste
- 1 tablespoon non dairy soy sour cream
- 2 tsp. arrowroot dissolved

Brown the spices in a non-stick pan. Then, in the food processor, put cashews, rice tomatoes and herbs. Bring the mixture to boil and simmer 5 or 6 minutes. Add arrowroot (dissolved) and non-dairy soy sour cream. Mix well.

PIZZA SAUCE

- 1 can tomatoes or crushed cooked fresh tomatoes
- 1 tablespoon dried onions
- 1 tomattia
- 1 green pepper chopped fine
- 1/2 cup mushrooms (cut in small slices)
- 1/2 cup seitan chopped
- 1/2 teaspoon chili powder
- 1/2 teaspoon paprika
- 1 teaspoon chopped parsley
- 1 pinch each basil, oregano, lemon thyme, dill weed
- 1 tablespoon concentrated apple juice
- 1/2 teaspoon garlic paste

Brown all herbs and garlic paste in dry non-stick pan for a short time, stirring all of the time. Squeeze 1/8 tsp. lemon juice on top.

Simmer 22 minutes. If you need sauce to be thicker, add 1-1/2 teaspoon dissolved arrowroot.

Entres

KABOBS PER 1 SKEWER

Marinate ingredients first, but be sure they do not become mushy. Put on skewer.

- 1 small mushroom
- 1 slice of green pepper
- Baby zucchini
- 1 thin small chunk of eggplant
- Small Roma tomatoes marinated (make 3 small holes in pack of tomatoes before marinating)

Keep adding tomato, zucchini, eggplant, pineapple (1 slice of unsweetened pineapple) until skewer is filled. See marinade.

Other vegetables to use are all kinds of sweet peppers, steamed artichokes, steamed asparagus tips, etc. Apples, pears, apricots and pineapples can be used (See fruit marinade).

Another kabob could be mushrooms, cherry tomato, sweet peppers and soy wieners cut into chunks. Or chicken (of course, vegetarian chicken) cut into chunks, or mushrooms and tomatoes are great. Use barbecue sauce without added oil or preservatives.

When you marinate, observe so that nothing becomes soggy.

Marinade for vegetables:
- 3 tablespoons of herb vinegar (like thyme vinegar, etc)
- 1 tablespoon fruit vinegar (sweet)
- 1 tsp. garlic paste
- 1/4 teaspoon onion powder

If you use herb vinegar, for example vinegar with a sprig of thyme, use also a pinch of thyme in your marinade. Baste several times while cooking. For fruit marinade use berry vinegars, for example blackberry or strawberry or raspberry vinegar.

Add some crushed berries like 1 or 2 to each fruit you are making into a kabob. You can have all fruit or all vegetable kebobs, or you can mix them, or serve 1 fruit and 1 vegetable kabob.

Baste the veggie meat, or chicken wieners with barbecue sauce that does not have added sugar, no preservatives. You can add 1/2 teaspoon to 1 cup of liquid smoke flavor, turn and baste often. Garlic and onion powder will make the barbecue sauce more delicious.

If you don't have a grill, lay filled skewers in a long pan. Keep basting and turning often. Bake at 350 to 375 degrees until almost tender. Serve with a small dish of chutney (a fruit for the fruits).

RAVIOLI (that you can make from scratch)

Pasta dough

- 2-2/3 cup whole-wheat pastry flour
- 1 tsp. crushed dill weed
- 2 tablespoons olive oil
- About 1/2 cup water

Mix everything together but the water. Add water only a little at a time or put everything into a food processor for about 1-1/2 minutes until workable dough is formed.

Knead by hand (add more flour if needed) Knead until dough is smooth. Roll dough into two sheets. Stretch the dough out. Put filling on top of one sheet of dough. Cover with the other sheet, cut into individual bite size squares. Pinch squares top and bottom sides together.

Drop raviolis in boiling water. Nudge raviolis with plastic or wooden spoon. Cook for about 8 or 10 minutes.

Serve with a no fat pasta sauce, a dab of soy sour cream fresh ground parsley. Steam kale and puree filling well in a food processor or use pureed spinach.

- 2 pinches each nutmeg, parsley, and allspice (spices ground).
- 1/4 cup no-dairy cheese
- 1-1/2 teaspoon dissolved arrowroot
- Garlic and onion to taste

Puree kale or spinach in food processor, add all herbs and seasonings and mix well with dissolved arrowroot. Fill ravioli dough.

Variation:

-Add to above
- 2 tablespoons non-dairy soy sour cream
- 1 tablespoon chopped chives

FRENCH NOODLES
- 1 lb. noodles (rice, whole wheat, soy, etc., but no white flour, or egg noodles)
- Do not add salt to water (you do not need the added sodium!)
- 1/4 cup soy sour cream (non dairy)
- 1/2 cup parsley ground very finely
- 1 tablespoon olive oil
- 1/4 cup non dairy cheese
- Garlic and onion powder to taste
- 2 teaspoons arrowroot power dissolved
- 1/2 cup sliced mushrooms
- Cook spaghetti. Do not use salt in the water, drain well.

- Brown mushrooms with 1 teaspoon olive oil.
- Heat half of soy sour cream, stir in half of the non-dairy cheese, garlic and onion powder to taste. Add the remainder of the olive oil and the dissolved arrowroot.
- Keep stirring – keep heat low. When warm and thick, pour over drained warm noodles; add mushrooms (also warm). Mix gently until noodles are well coated. Sprinkle with ground parsley. Garnish with a sprig of parsley.

SPAGHETTI ITALIAN

- 3/4 lb. of good spaghetti (artichoke, rice, whole wheat, soy, etc., but no white flour, or egg spaghetti)
- 1/2 cup of white home made no-dairy cheese
- 4 green onion bottoms, finely minced
- 1 cup sauce (no fat)
- 1 cup teaspoon garlic paste
- 1 teaspoon paprika (not hot kind)
- 1/4 teaspoon each: crushed dried basil, crushed dried dill and 1 tablespoon of ground rye parsley
- Garlic and onion powder to taste
- 1/2 lb. of fresh mushrooms, cleaned and sliced

Cook spaghetti. Brown onion bottoms and garlic paste. Add mushrooms and all herbs. Brown in olive oil, add sauce and half of all the cheese. Heat until everything is well heated and blended. Add the rest of non-dairy cheese. Garnish with fresh parsley.

EGGPLANT ITALIAN

Cut eggplant thin. Bake on cookie sheet and brush with olive oil. Broil until soft enough to roll up with filling.

Filling

- Fresh mint
- Dried tomatoes in olive oil
- Non-dairy homemade cheese
- Artichoke hearts (all chopped)

Roll up into eggplant roll. Sprinkle with non-dairy cheese. Put in a greased dish. Bake at 350 degrees for about 20 minutes. Garnish with freshly chopped mint.

RUSSIAN/POLISH PEROGI

- 5 cups pastry whole wheat flour
- 1 package or 1 tablespoon baking yeast
- 1 tablespoon unsweetened frozen pineapple concentrate (no sugar type)
- 1/4 cup warm water (not boiling)
- 3/4 cup low fat soy milk
- 1 tablespoon and 1 teaspoon olive oil

Dissolve yeast in water with pineapple juice. Let stand until yeast bubbles, fizzes. Add 2-1/2 cups of flour to soymilk and olive oil. Stir in yeast. Put dough on board, add more flour and knead for 5-to-6 minutes. Dough should be elastic. Allow dough to rise and punch down. Cut out rounds 4 inches across.

Filling
(You may wish to double filling)

- 3/4 lb. fresh mushrooms sliced
- 2 slices whole wheat bread (no preservatives, fat)
- 1-1/2 tsp. dried onions
- 1/2 teaspoon garlic paste
- 1/2 teaspoon dried crushed dill weed
- 1/2 teaspoon parsley dried
- 1/4 cup seitan finely chopped
- 1 1/2 teaspoon olive oil

Brown breaded mushrooms. Place everything (except olive oil which has already been used) in with browned mushrooms: bread and herbs. Mix well, fill perogies. Bake at 350-degrees.

Alternate Cabbage Filling
- 2 cups finely shredded cabbage (packed well)
- 2 tsp. dried dill weed- 4 bottoms green onions minced
- 2 tablespoons non-dairy cheese
- 2 tsp. ground caraway seeds

- 1 tablespoon olive oil

Brown green onions and herbs. Add non-dairy cheese. Put into center of dough.

NON-MEAT MEATBALL ENTREES
- 1/4 cup rice milk
- 2 cups whole wheat ground flour
- 3 tablespoons dried onions
- 3/4 cup good vegetable stock (see recipe under misc.)
- 1 tablespoon low sodium soy sauce
- 1/4 teaspoon each oregano, dill weed, parsley, lemon thyme
- 1/4 teaspoon garlic paste
- 2 tablespoons fine whole wheat bread crumbs
- 1 tablespoon non-dairy soy sour cream
- 1/4 potato flour

Mix well. Roll into balls. (If too moist, add more potato flour). Bake on a non-stick cookie sheet at 350-degrees for about 20 minutes. Turn once so they are cooked on all sides. Use in spaghetti and any other meatball dishes.

Variations: Served cooked in mushroom sauce or pasta sauce or brown gravy or sweet-and-sour sauce.

LATINO BLACK BEANS AND SAFRON RICE
- 2 large cans (or 3 cups dried beans, cooked)
- 1/4 tsp. garlic paste
- 1-1/2 tsp. ground cumin
- 2 teaspoons dried ground dill weed
- 2 teaspoons dried onions
- 2 teaspoons dried ground parsley
- 3/4 teaspoon lemon thyme
- 1 tablespoon lime juice plus peel zest of 1/2 lime
- 1 large sweet green pepper chopped
- 1 large or 1-1/2 medium chopped sweet red pepper
- 1/2 teaspoon sweet (not hot) paprika
- 1/4 teaspoon mild chili (ground)
- 3/4 cup no fat spaghetti sauce
- 1 tsp. coconut flavor

- 1/2 tsp. grated ginger (fresh and peeled)

Add everything but limejuice to cooked beans. Simmer everything until well blended. Just before serving, add the limejuice. Serve over saffron rice with a thin slice/ twist of fresh lime.

PERSIAN LENTILS (adas pelo)

- 1-1/2 cups brown rice cooked
- 1 cup seedless raisins
- 1/4 cup pitted chopped dates (well washed)
- 2 bottoms, green onions cut fine
- 3/4 lb. seitan (1 package)
- 3/4 cup lentils cooked
- 1 teaspoon ground mint
- 1/4 cup berry vinegar

Brown, cut seitan into pan (stirring constantly), add cooked lentils, chopped pitted dates. In pan layer cooked rice, lentils, seitan, raisins and dates. Add berry vinegar, cover. Cook until everything is warm. Garnish with ground mint.

MOCK OYSTERS ON THE SHELL

To make mock oysters, use oyster mushrooms. Clean, cut off large stems (save to use at another time). Steam oyster mushrooms slightly. Add a few pinches of finely ground nori and a pinch of garlic powder to the olive oil. Brush mushrooms lightly with the olive oil concoction. Garnish with a touch of Hungarian paprika and a sprinkle of finely ground parsley. Serve in a shell.

CHINESE MOCK SWEET AND SOUR PORK

Make sweet-and-sour sauce first and put aside.

- 2 parts of white rice vinegar
- 2 parts no fat pasta sauce
- 1/2 part low sodium soy sauce
- 2 parts water
- 1 part frozen-concentrated pineapple juice
- 2 teaspoon arrowroot dissolved

Bring all ingredients to a boil. Thicken with dissolved arrowroot.

To make the mock pork, use vegetarian ground chicken roll 1/2 cup.

- 3/4 teaspoon fresh ground ginger.
- 1/2 teaspoon liquid smoke flavor
- 1 teaspoon bacon yeast.

Follow directions for non-fat meatballs. After baking meatballs, pour all but 2 tablespoons of the sweet and sour sauce over them and add:

- 1/4 to 1/2 cup unsweetened canned pineapple, cut into chunks
- 1/4 cup green peppers
- 1/4 cup red pepper

Heat well and serve with 2 tablespoons of sweet-and-sour sauce poured over the top.

MUSHROOM BALLS

- 2-1/4 cups washed and chopped fresh mushrooms, any kind
- 2 cups dry bread crumbs (healthy bread)
- 6 tablespoons potato flour
- 1/2 teaspoon ground dried parsley
- 1/4 teaspoon dill weed dried crumbled
- 1/4 teaspoon lemon thyme
- 1 tablespoon dried onions
- 2 tablespoons fresh parsley (ground) as garnish
- 1 tablespoon soy sour cream. (Non dairy)
- Garlic powder to taste

Use enough mushroom juice to form balls (can be omitted). Mix everything together. Shape into balls with hands. Bake at 350-degrees on non-stick cookie sheet. Turn once. Serve with mushroom gravy. Garnish with fresh ground parsley.

SLOPPY JOES

(Use barbecue type of seitan or plain seitan)

- 1 cup of seitan (ground like burger)
- 2 tablespoons dried onions
- 3/4 tsp. garlic paste
- 1/2 cup finely chopped green sweet pepper
- 1/2 cup pasta sauce
- 1/4 cup pickle water
- 2 teaspoon (no alum, no preservative, chopped pickles

Mix, put into greased non-stick pan. Bake at 350-degrees for 20-25 minutes. Serve on whole wheat buns (100 % whole wheat, no preservatives, no oil) with lettuce, tomato and pasta sauce and pickles. Or serve as an entree with baked potatoes or hash browns, cooked without oil.

NO OIL HASH-BROWN POTATOES

Peel and shred raw potatoes. Make little mountains of raw shredded potatoes on a non-stick greased cookie sheet. Bake at 400-degrees until potatoes are cooked Turn potatoes.

BELGIUM SPINACH ARTICHOKE CASSEROLE

- 7 ounces homemade marinated artichoke hearts
- 1/2 lb. mushrooms sliced
- 1/2 teaspoon garlic paste
- 10 ounces lightly steamed spinach
- 1/4 cup non dairy sour cream
- 1/2 teaspoon ground nutmeg
- 1 pinch ground dill
- 1/2 teaspoon lime juice
- 1/2 teaspoon lemon juice
- Pine nuts for garnish
- Pimiento strips for garnish

Put the artichoke marinade into a pan. Cook mushrooms, add garlic paste and stir constantly, remove from heat. The spinach should be shredded and gently steamed until almost wilted. Add spinach, nutmeg, dill, lemon and limejuice. Add half of the non-dairy sour cream, all herbs and seasonings and mix gently and well. Put into greased casserole dish. Bake at 350-degrees for 10 minutes. Garnish with dabs of the non-dairy sour cream, pine nuts and pimiento. This is great for special occasions.

MOCK PRAWNS

- 3 medium sized red potatoes (peeled and grated)
- 1/2 cup potato flour
- 1/8 cup rice milk
- 2 small French carrots peeled, slightly steamed and grated
- 3 tablespoons mock tuna, defrosted and crumbled
- 1 teaspoon ground nori
- 2 teaspoon arrowroot dissolved

Mix everything together. Shape into prawn-like shapes. Dip in rice milk – then into potato flour.

Place on a greased sheet non-stick cookie sheet. Bake at 350-degrees, turn once. Serve in cocktail sauce (see recipe in sauces) or with saffron rice.

NON-EGG FOO YOUNG (no dairy, no eggs)

- 1-1/2 cups rice flour
- 1 tablespoon dried onions
- 1 cup fresh bean sprouts
- 1 tablespoon soy sauce (low sodium)
- 1 tablespoon green onion tops finely chopped
- 1 teaspoon arrowroot dissolved
- 2/3 cup low-fat hard tofu
- 1 teaspoon grated ginger

Put everything into a food processor except the green onion tops and bean sprouts. Allow batter to stand 5 to 6 minutes. Drop onto non-stick cookie sheet and bake at 350 degrees. Turn once. Brown on both sides.

Pour very hot water over bean sprouts, then very cold water. Steam for one minute only. The bean sprouts should just turn white and be crunchy. Drain, place on top of each Foo Young; sprinkle with a touch of ginger on top. Roll up and serve.

ROCKERFELLER OYSTERS (MUSHROOMS)

- 8 ounces oyster mushrooms (fresh)
- 2 tablespoons no-fat soy sour cream

- 1 teaspoon capers
- 1 teaspoon lemon juice
- Garlic and onion (one pinch of each)
- 1 teaspoon finely chopped nori

Mix everything but the mushrooms together, chill well. Slightly steam the oyster mushrooms that have been gently cleaned and chilled.

Chill. Mix mushrooms gently in part of the Rockefeller mixture. Arrange mushrooms in individual oyster shells.

Place shells on chopped ice. Serve fresh lemon slices on chopped ice. The oyster mushrooms must not be drowned in Rockefeller dressing so it's a good idea to place the other half of the Rockefeller dressing in a bowl on the ice. Allow the oyster mushrooms to be seen.

HUNGARIAN NOODLES

- 1 lb. spaghetti or noodles (Hungarians use noodles rather than spaghetti). Be certain to use healthy pasta. No white flour, no eggs or dairy.
- 2 tablespoons Japanese rice vinegar, no seasoning
- 1 teaspoon each lemon juice and lime juice
- 2 tablespoons non-dairy cheese
- 1/8 cup soysauce (low sodium)
- 1 tablespoon non-dairy sour cream
- 1 teaspoon olive oil
- 1-1/2 teaspoons paprika
- 1 tablespoon green onion (cut very fine)
- 1/4 teaspoon lemon thyme (crushed fine)
- 1/4 teaspoon dried basil (crushed)
- 1/4 teaspoon dried mint (crushed)
- 1/8 teaspoon dried rosemary (crushed)
- Use sweet peppers (1 large yellow pepper or 2 large red peppers and 1/2 green pepper)

Cook spaghetti and drain (Do not use salt in water). Brown herbs and peppers in olive oil. Mix noodles with vinegar, lemon and limejuices.

Cover, simmer. In a bowl put soy sour cream, garlic and onion powder to taste mix well. Garnish with paprika and dabs of soy sour cream.

"KHORESH – EFERENJAN" A Persian dish

- 2/3 cups bread crumbs
- 2 bottoms green onions, grated
- 1/2 lb. shelled ground walnuts
- 1/2 lb. ground seitan (like hamburger)
- 1/2 cup pomegranate juice concentrate
- Garlic and onion powder to taste
- 1 teaspoon olive oil
- Grind walnuts until they are like coarse corn meal
- Brown rice

Brown onion bottoms in olive oil. Add breadcrumbs and crushed walnuts. Stir constantly. Do not burn, add crumbled seitan.

Add 1/4 cup hot water, 1/2 pomegranate juice. Cover and let simmer add rest of pomegranate juice. Stir well. Add garlic and onion powder. Serve over brown rice. This is a rich dish – just a taste or two. Eat sparingly.

PACIFIC RIM STIR FRY (serve hot over saffron brown rice)

- 2/3 cups bread crumbs
- 2 bottoms green onions, grated
- 1/2 lb. shelled walnuts
- 1/2 lb. ground seitan (like hamburger)
- 1/2 cup pomegranate juice concentrate (you must use pomegranate juice in this dish) concentrated form without sugar or preservatives). You can also juice your own fresh pomegranate.
- 1/2 cup hot water
- Garlic and onion powder to taste
- 1 teaspoon olive oil
- Grind walnuts until they are like coarse corn meal
- 1/2 lb. oriental peas in pods
- 1/2 lb. thin string beans, green or yellow, slightly steamed quite crunchy
- 1/3 cup green onion tops (chopped fine)
- 2 large green peppers
- 1 large red pepper
- 1 large yellow pepper
- 1–1/2 oriental eggplant
- 1/4 cup steamed cauliflower

- 1/2 tsp. garlic paste
- 1/4 cup broccoli
- 1 cup sprouts (blanched)
- 1/2 lb. fresh mushrooms sliced
- 1–1/2 tsp. chopped chives
- 1–1/2 cups Chinese cabbage (nappa) shredded
- 1 tiny bunch baby (only) bok choy
- 2 tablespoons melon or pineapple (fresh if possible – no sugar added)
- 1 tablespoon olive oil
- 2 tsp. low sodium soy sauce
- 2 tablespoons peeled ground ginger
- 2 tsp. arrowroot dissolved
- 1 tablespoon apple concentrate

Brown onion bottoms in olive oil, add eggplant, the peppers, vegetables. Lastly the sprouts. If too dry, add 1 tablespoon homemade vegetable stock or Miso broth diluted in water. Garnish with green onion tops.

BAKED FELAFEL

- 2 cups of chickpeas (garbanzo beans, canned).
- 3/4 teaspoon garlic paste
- 1 teaspoon dried onions
- 1/2 teaspoon ground cumin
- 1 teaspoon tahini
- 2+ beads of saffron separated
- 3 tablespoons potato flour

Put drained chickpeas in food processor. Run food processor until chickpeas are a soft paste. Combine all the ingredients except potato flour. Make small (flat) patties.

Bake on a greased non-stick cookie sheet 350-degrees; turn once. Serve with tahini lemon lime sauce thinly, place sliced peeled cucumbers on top.

Sauce

- 1 tablespoon tahini
- 1/2 tablespoon of soy non-dairy sour cream
- 1 teaspoon each of lime juice and lemon juice (fresh)
- 2 tablespoons soy milk (garlic and onion powder to taste)
- 1 teaspoon ground cumin

- 1/2 teaspoon each ground mint, ground parsley and whisk well
- 2 teaspoon arrowroot (dissolved); whisk again

BROCCOLI CASSEROLE

- 2 cups of broccoli (flowers, small part of stems)
- 2 ounces of chopped pimientos
- 1 cup of bread crumbs (good whole wheat, no preservatives)
- 1 cup cooked mushrooms
- 1/4 cup soy sour cream
- 1/4 cup white soy non dairy cheese

Steam broccoli (keep crisp and green). Put into a casserole dish; add 1/2 soy sour cream, onion and garlic powder to taste

Add 1/2 pimientos, cooked mushrooms. Mix well. Add breadcrumbs and non-dairy cheese to the top of the mixture. Bake 350-degrees, serve hot with chopped parsley, pimiento (sliced) and dab of soy sour cream.

VEGGIE LOAF

- 1-1/2 cups cooked millet (soft, mashed with rice milk)
- 1-1/2 cups cooked brown rice
- 2 cups dry bread crumbs (no oil or preservatives)
- 1-1/2 cups Napa cabbage shredded (slightly steamed and mashed)
- 1 cup shredded onions
- 3/4 cup non-dairy soy cream
- Garlic and onion powder to taste
- 8 tablespoons potato or Spelt flour
- 1/2 tablespoon concentrated (frozen) apple juice (measure while frozen)
- 1/4 cup baked or boiled potatoes, mashed
- 2 small jars of pimientos
- 1/2 cup tomato sauce, no fat
- 1/2 teaspoon each oregano, marjoram, dill weed, parsley, sage
- 1/8 teaspoon saffron

Blend all ingredients in food processor. Add potato or Spelt flour to hold the loaf together. Put in a non-stick greased bread pan.

Bake at 350-degrees until chopstick put into center of loaf comes out clean 1/2 way through. Garnish with 1/2 of the tomato sauce and top with ground fresh parsley.

Variation: Fresh (cooked) mushroom gravy or white sauce is good too.

CORN TORTILLAS WITH SOUR CHUTNEY

- 8 corn tortillas
- 3 fresh bananas
- 4 tsp. fresh non dairy cheese
- 4 tablespoons non-sweet chutney like lime ginger, tomato chutney etc.

Put each corn tortilla (already made) into a dry non-stick pan and heat on each side until tortillas are soft and bend easily. Cut fresh bananas thinly and lengthwise.

Put 3/4 tsp. of non-dairy cheese in the center of each tortilla. Heat in non-stick baking dish. Be careful that the tortillas do not get hard.

Cook only until tortilla is warm and cheese is mushy. Serve with a tiny dish of chutney so each person can use what he or she wants of chutney over the tortillas.

VARIATION: Instead of bananas use other fruits 1/4 teaspoon chutney. I like bananas the best for this dish.

INDIAN PAKORAS (VEGETABLE FRITTERS)
NOT fried - they are BAKED

- 2 cups chick pea flour
- 4 tablespoons very cold water
- 1/4 tsp. ground cumin
- 1/8 tsp. ground cardamom
- 1 inch of saffron (crush it a bit)
- 1/4 cup cooked diced mushrooms
- 1/8 cup ground fresh parsley
- 1/8 cup ground tops of green onions finely chopped.
- 1/2 of a banana sliced.

Mix a small potato and one oriental eggplant peeled, cooked and mashed together.

Mix batter together. (Dough must not have any lumps. Stir in mushrooms, bananas, eggplant/potato.

Form into small balls. Bake in 350-degree oven on an oiled non-stick cookie sheet. Turn once. Brown on both sides (it should be cooked all around and inside). Garnish with onion tops.

Variation: Leftover mashed potatoes are good as a filling. Also mashed sweet potatoes or yams (steamed ahead of time) or baked mashed yellow squash. If using squash or sweet potatoes or yams, add one pinch of cinnamon, allspice and nutmeg.

BARBECUE VEGETABLE ROLL

Spread a thin touch of humus dip and barbecue sauce on large oil free chapatti or corn tortilla (must be very large).

Add roasted peeled peppers, eggplant (cut into thin strips) and tomato slices. Add a sprinkle of sesame seeds. Roll up halfway; add ground parsley finish rolling up. Serve with sprigs of parsley.

BABA GANOUSH/BABA GHANNOUJ ROLLUPS

- 2 tablespoons homemade hummus spread with teaspoon olive oil
- 1-1/2 tablespoons barbecue sauce (without added oil, sugar or preservatives)
- 1 large red pepper (roasted and peeled)
- 1-1/2 green pepper (roasted and peeled)
- 3/4 yellow pepper (roasted and peeled)
- 2 Japanese eggplant (peeled and roasted)
- Alfalfa sprouts
- 1-1/2 tomato
- Ground parsley
- Sesame seeds
- One whole wheat chapatti, pita, or large tortilla (no added oil or preservatives) for each roll-up.

- 2 tsp. parsley (ground)
- 1 pinch ground cumin powder
- 2 tsp. homemade baba ganoush
- 1 tsp. dried onions
- 1 tsp. very finely chopped green onion tops (cut onions very finely)
- Zest 1/2 small lemon
- 1/2 tsp. fresh lemon juice
- Spread baba ganoush on the chapatti, pita bread or light corn tortilla
- Next a pinch of ground cumin
- Finely ground parsley
- 1 teaspoon fine dried onions
- A sprinkle of alfalfa sprouts

Pit and pulverize the dates, add on top of the Baba ganoush or just under the sprouts. Sprinkle dates with lemon juice. Roll up and garnish with lemon zest.

SPINACH LENTIL LOAF ENTREE
- 1/2 cup spinach pureed
- 1-1/2 cup lentils
- 1 tablespoon dried onions
- 1 bay leaf
- 1/2 cup rice milk
- 3/4 cup fine bread crumbs (bread no preservatives)
- 1/2 teaspoon cumin (ground)
- 1/2 teaspoon rosemary (ground)
- 1/4 teaspoon nutmeg
- 1/8 teaspoon fine, dried mint (ground)
- Garlic powder to taste
- 1/2 red pepper sliced for garnish

Cook lentils with a bay leaf. Remove bay leaf after it is cooked. Spinach can be steamed slightly.

Puree the spinach, breadcrumbs, herbs, lentils etc. in food processor. Add rice milk and mix well. Bake in a greased non-stick loaf pan at 350-degrees for about 45 minutes. When top is slightly brown, cover. Garnish with sliced red peppers. Can be served hot or cold.

Variation: Serve with gravy or can be eaten cold with a dipping sauce.

NON-DAIRY CHEESE ROLL UP

For one roll up:
- Large chapatti or tortilla (no oil)
- 1 teaspoon non-dairy white cheese
- Pimiento non-dairy cheese
- Tomatoes (sliced thin)
- Juice of 1/2 of a fresh lime
- 1 teaspoon grated zest lime
- 1 slice fresh melon
- 2 slices fresh banana

Melt non-dairy pimiento cheese and spread over tortilla large or chapatti. Place the fruit in the chapatti or tortilla and add 1/2 of the limejuice.

Put the tomato slices on the chapatti and add the non-dairy cheese. Heat just until non-dairy cheese starts to melt. Serve hot. Garnish with a sprinkle of lime zest.

ARTICHOKE EXTRAORDINARE

- 6 large artichokes
- 1-1/4 lb. mushrooms
- 1 tsp. garlic paste
- Onion powder to taste
- 1 tablespoons white non dairy cheese
- 1 teaspoon rice vinegar
- 1 tablespoon fresh parsley ground
- 2 teaspoons arrowroot dissolved
- 1 cup (good homemade vegetable stock or 1-1/2 cups miso (already diluted)

Cook cored artichokes with cleaned mushrooms (add mushrooms later as it takes less time for the mushrooms to cook than the artichokes).

When done put the mushrooms in the food processor with the garlic paste and the onion powder etc. Make into a paste fill the artichokes (center of artichoke that has been scooped out) with the mushrooms.

Put the miso and artichoke mushroom juice in a baking pan and heat (in the juice), the stuffed artichoke. Dab with vinegar on top of the artichoke. Cover. Bake.

Add the dissolved arrowroot to juice and continue baking for a few minutes until the arrowroot thickens a bit. Serve warm with sauce poured over the artichoke and grown parsley on top.

NEW ORLEANS HOT WEATHER VEGIE CHICKEN ENTREE

- Sage 2 pinches
- Pinch each of oregano nutmeg, garlic and onion powder to taste
- Juice of one juicy lime
- 1/4 cup raisins
- 1 cup frozen veggie chicken roll cut into chunks
- 1/2 can unsweetened pineapple chunks
- 1-1/2 teaspoons olive oil
- 1 teaspoon natural coconut flavor mixed with soy non-dairy sour cream.

Brown the veggie chicken chunks in the olive oil. Brown the herbs add small amount of juice from pineapple.

Add raisins, pineapple, coconut flavor and mixed soy sour cream last. Arrange on a platter with a few chunks of pineapple and raisins as a garnish.

GINGER SOY ENTREE

For one roll up

- Large whole wheat chapatti (without added oil or fat or preservatives, or large corn tortilla)
- 1/4/ to 1/2 tsp low fat tofu soy cream
- 1 teaspoon grated ginger
- 1 large stalk of lemon grass (pounded)
- 1/4 juice fresh lemon an 1/2 zest lemon
- 1-1/2 slices pineapple crushed
- 1/2 teaspoon nutmeg

Marinate ginger in homemade soy sour cream and the finely ground nutmeg for at least 2 hours in refrigerator. Spread soy cream on large chapatti or large corn tortilla. Drop the fresh lemon juice on the pineapple

Lay the pounded lemon grass over the tortilla or chapatti. Let stand for 1/2 hour. Remove the lemon grass. (roll up the roll-up). Use the lemon grass as a garnish and sprinkle with lemon zest. Do not allow the roll-up to get soggy.

STROGANOFF ENTREE

- 1 lb. fresh mushrooms
- 1/2 cup seitan cut into small pieces
- 2 bottoms of green tops minced finely
- 3/4 lb. Whole wheat noodles (wide noodles)
- 1 tablespoon ground fresh parsley
- 1/2 cup soy sour cream (homemade)
- 1 pinch dill weed crumbled
- 1/2 tsp. garlic paste
- 1 tsp. olive oil
- 3/4 tablespoon Balsamic vinegar
- Garlic and onion powder to taste

Clean and cut mushrooms. Mash and puree bottoms of green onions in non-stick pan. Brown onions and mushrooms and herbs in oil. Add vinegar, seitan and soy sour cream last.

Cook whole-wheat noodles. Drain well. Mix in with rest of above ingredients. Garnish with sprinkle of ground parsley and a dribble of sweet paprika.

SWEET AND SOUR GRAPE LEAVES

- Soak grape leaves for several hours. (change the water several times)
- Soak green olives, do the same as with grape leaves and remove as much salt as possible
- Wash brown rice well
- Add onions, dill weed, figs, olives and mix with the rice
- Wrap the grape leaves around the mixture

Cook in already heated tomatoes. Top with thin slivers of white non-dairy cheese. Garnish with the rest of the ground parsley and chopped green olives

CREPES LA BONNE FEMME

- 1 lb. fresh mushrooms
- 1/2 cup seitan cut into small pieces
- 2 bottoms of green tops minced finely
- 3/4 lb. whole wheat noodles (wide whole wheat or rice noodles)
- 1 tablespoon ground fresh parsley
- 1/2 cup low fat soy sour cream (homemade)
- 1 pinch dill weed crumbled
- 1/2 tsp. garlic paste
- 1 teaspoon olive oil
- 3/4 tablespoon balsamic vinegar
- Garlic and onion powder to taste

BATTER

- 1-3/4 cup soy milk (lowfat)
- 1/2 cup homemade soy cream
- 1 cup rice flour
- 1/4 cup raw cashews (pieces)
- 1 tsp. dry soy milk powder

Blend everything in food processor. The cashews must be like a fine butter, no lumps.

FILLING

Puree 1 package of defrosted spinach.

- 2 tablespoons non dairy white cheese
- 1 tsp. nutmeg (ground)
- 1 tablespoon non dairy soy cream

Use a nonstick pan (grease) pour crepes quite thin. Turn out filling into center of crepes. Garnish with a sprinkle of finely ground parsley.

CHINESE MOCK FISH

- 1 package firm fat free bean curd/tofu
- 4 to 6 ounces mashed potatoes
- 1/2 teaspoon smoke flavor
- 2 teaspoons dissolved arrowroot

- 1-1/2 tablespoons olive oil
- 1/2 roll vegetarian defrosted tuna roll
- Sheets of nori (sea weed)

Mash soy bean curd with mashed potatoes, mashed defrosted mock tuna roll. Add smoke flavor. Shape into fish cutlets. Wrap strips of nori around the cutlets Brush nori lightly with olive oil.

Place on greased nonstick cookie sheet. Broil until lightly browned on both sides. Serve warm with ginger sauce.

GRILLED OR BROILED PORTABELLO MUSHROOMS

- Large portabella mushrooms
- 3/4 tablespoon olive oil
- 1 tablespoon finely ground fresh parsley
- Garlic and onion powder to taste

Wash portabella mushrooms. Broil or grill and (turn once)
Mix olive oil with onion, garlic powder and 1/2 ground parsley. Pour over the grilled or broiled portabella. Garnish with ground parsley

Variation: 3/4 tablespoon unsalted pine nuts.
Cut up 3/4 cup ripe, peeled and seeded papaya Heat the fruit and pine nuts and add to the cooked portabella.

ASIAN ISLAND VEGETARIAN CHICKEN

- 3/4 cup thinly chopped green onions
- 1/4 cup raisins
- 1/4 cup chopped black figs
- 2 cups cooked brown basmati rice (precook with two threads of saffron)
- 1/4 cup cashew nuts (unsalted) pieces
- 1/2 frozen chicken roll (chopped)
- 1 pinch each cumin powder, sage
- 2 teaspoons olive oil
- 1 tablespoon unsalted roasted peanuts
- 1/2 cup rice milk
- 1/2 to 1 tsp. good pure coconut flavor
- 1/2 tsp. curry powder

Brown onions in olive oil add herbs, raisins and figs. Defrost veggie chicken, cut into long strips and sprinkle with curry powder.

Use only drops at a time of the rice milk to which has been added coconut flavor. Use rice milk sparingly only to keep the ingredients from burning.

Mix everything gently, but well. Put rice at the bottom of a nonstick pan that has been greased. Mound rest of recipe on top. Bake for 20 to 25 minutes at 350 degrees. Garnish with the chopped peanuts and lime slices. Serve with chutney.

VEGIE CHICKEN LOAF

- 1/2 cup of veggie (frozen) chicken roll, ground fine
- 1 tablespoon dried onions
- 1 teaspoon garlic paste
- 1 tablespoon ground fresh parsley
- 1/2 cup cooked brown basmati rice
- 1/2 cup soy milk
- 1/8 cup of pine nuts or unsalted cashews (chopped coarsely)
- 1 pinch each sage, rosemary, cardamom (all crumpled very fine)
- 1/2 cup whole wheat or seven grain finely crumpled bread crumbs
- 2 tablespoons white non-dairy cheese

Use a food processor, add brown rice and run until rice becomes a very smooth ball. Combine everything in processor run just a couple of times. Be sure that everything is well mixed. Pour in the soymilk a little at a time.

Put into a non-stick greased loaf pan. Bake at 350 degrees for about one hour. If you want it real firm you can bake it a little longer.

A chopstick stuck in the center than comes out clean shows you it is done. Garnish with parsley sprig. Serve with chutney. See chutney recipe.

UNUSUAL VEGGIE CHICKEN (EASY RECIPE)

- 1/4 to 1/2 roll of vegetarian chicken—defrosted
- 1/4 cup unsweetened pineapple juice
- 1 cup of green cabbage (no core) shredded and packed solidly

- 1/2 cup homemade Thousand Island dressing (see recipe under salad dressings)

Slice defrosted roll of veggie chicken into round slices. Place on non-stick pan add pineapple juice and top chicken slices with 1/8 cup of Thousand Island dressing. Put the shredded cabbage on top of the Thousand Island dressing.

Add the rest of the Thousand Island dressing all over the top of the cabbage. Cover. Bake at 350 degrees, when hot and tender serve.

CHOP SUEY WITH NOODLES

- 1 package buckwheat Japanese noodles
- 6 stalks celery, finely chopped
- 1 green pepper sliced very thin
- 2 red peppers sliced very thin
- 6 tablespoons Bamboo shoots sliced very thin
- 2 cups fresh bean sprouts
- 1/2 cup good homemade vegetable stock
- 1 package teriyaki seitan (cut into small pieces)
- 1 tablespoon miniature corn
- 1-1/2 tablespoons teriyaki sauce
- 1/4 cup unsweetened pineapple juice
- 1 tablespoon arrowroot, dissolved
- 1/2 package bean threads (like spaghetti)
- 6 pre-soaked black mushrooms (steam them until quite soft)
- 1 tablespoon Japanese vinegar
- 1/2 tsp. grated ginger

Cook noodles, drain and add to all above ingredients. Add bean thread noodles last and spread them out as you put it into the pan. Cook until vegetables are crunchy. Garnish with finely cut strips of nori.

Variation: Can use veggie chicken roll cut into small slices (strips) instead of seitan.

CHICKEN A' LA KING
- 1/2 cup of red peppers
- 4 bottoms of green onion, finely chopped and placed inside of the chicken roll (see recipe of stuffed veggie chicken)
- 1/2 teaspoon dried sage ground
- 1/2 teaspoon crushed rosemary ground
- 1 teaspoon parsley dried ground
- 1 pinch crushed dried mint
- 2 tablespoons pimientos (no liquid)
- 1-1/2 tsp. dissolved arrowroot
- 3/4 cup cleaned fresh chopped mushrooms
- 2 tablespoons (raw) cashew butter or 1 cup of raw cashews that are blended to a butter in the food processor
- 1/2 tsp. garlic paste
- 3/4 cup rice milk or soy milk (low fat)

Brown herbs, red peppers, mushrooms onion bottoms in non stick pan. Add rice milk or soy sauce a little at a time, veggie chicken.

Simmer, add cashew butter and dissolved arrowroot. Garnish with sprinkles of fresh ground parsley. Add a sprig of parsley as garnish.

DELUXE PIZZA
- 1-1/2 cups warm water
- 1 package dry yeast
- 2-1/2 cups whole wheat flour
- 1 tsp. concentrated canned frozen apple juice

Sprinkle yeast over apple juice in warm water. Wait until yeast foams. Mix everything together. Knead dough well. Let dough rise to double its size. Roll dough out.

Put dough on pizza pan (grease pan or dish keep dough thick. Spread with pizza sauce, (see recipe under sauces an gravy). Crumble non-dairy white cheese or any one of the following: Veggie Tuna roll crumbled, sliced vegetable chicken, marinated spiced tofu, etc.

Slice thin, add red, yellow and green peppers cut into strips and sliced slightly steamed mushrooms. Add 1/2 teaspoon chopped olives and 1/2 teaspoon capers. Add a sprinkle of ground parsley. Spread non-dairy white cheese on top (not too much non dairy-cheese). Bake at 400-degrees until crust is lightly brown.

VEGIE CHICKEN BREAD STUFFING

- Veggie chicken, hard tofu, or mushrooms (mushrooms &/or tofu should be browned with herbs). Crumble.
- 6 cups of toasted whole wheat bread cubes or French bread *without* preservatives, dairy or oil.
- 2 stalks of (white inside part) of celery, finely chopped
- 2 tablespoons dried onions
- 1/2 teaspoon garlic paste
- A pinch each dried rosemary sage, and parsley, crumbled
- Garlic and onion powder to taste
- 1 cup rice milk
- 2 teaspoons olive oil

Brown celery, onions and all the herbs in cubes of bread in olive oil.
Add rice milk. Bake in nonstick pan (cover pan).

Stir occasionally. Be careful that the dressing is not mushy. Stir in chopped (veggie) chicken roll. Sprinkle with fresh ground parsley and a sprinkle of paprika

STUFFED VEGGIE CHICKEN FOR THE HOLIDAYS

1 loaf of frozen veggie chicken roll or similar vegetarian meat substitute. Defrost it until it is easy to scoop out. Scoop out the center of roll. Make sure to keep veggie chicken that was scooped out on the side.

Add bread dressing to the center of the chicken. Add bread-dressing, pack tightly into chicken roll. Paint all around the roll of veggie chicken. Serve cranberry sauce.

Variation:

The bread stuffing can be heated on top of the stove. Stir constantly, add ground 1/8th cup walnuts. Stuff chicken roll. Heat stuffed veggie chicken in oven but do not cook. Serve cranberry relish on the side.

See recipes under gravy and sauce for both cranberry sauce and relish.

How to Make Good Tea

I remember one of my mother's good friends who was originally from England. Betty was always insisting that my mother should only make tea in the proper British manner. Eventually, my mother agreed and we will all benefit from Betty's traditional technique to also get all the nutrients from the herbal or real tea.

The first thing you need to remember is this – if you want a good pot of tea you must begin with quality tea. Poor quality tea will always make bad tea. Always start with quality tealeaves or tea sachets. Here are some guidelines:

- Start by using fresh, spring, or filtered water, and then add a level teaspoon of loose tea for every cup, plus one extra for the pot.

- Pre-heat the teapot by pouring boiling water into it and swishing it around, raising the temperature to 180° Fahrenheit. Discard the water.

- Next, add the tea by pouring boiling water over tea, which saturates the tea, producing a more flavorful extraction. Never add tea to hot water, as this will produce poor tea, because of the lower water temperature.

- Steeping Times: for black, white, oolong, and herbal teas -- steep at least 4-5 minutes. For green tea, use less than boiling water and steep 1-3 minutes. Place the lid on, and allow the tea to steep, covered.

- Strain and pour into a warmed teacup. It is said that most of us are unaware that you will enhance the flavor by serving tea in fine bone china or porcelain teacups. It results in a luxurious cup of tea. The Styrofoam cup from McDonalds just won't do it!

True British can serve black tea with milk and sugar. From a medical point of view, this is not an acceptable maneuver. If you must use 'white', use rice milk or almond milk. If you insist on sweet, use Stevia or honey.

Now that you have read this book, you will have the tools to start you on the road to implementing various strategies that WILL transform your health. This gentler approach to medicine will allow your body to heal and stimulate a more vibrant you. Enjoy the journey . . .

–Dr. Paul Davis

INDEX

Abhyanga, 25
ADHD, Attention Deficit
Hyperactivity Disorder, 80
Aging, 40–64
Agni, 25
Allergies, 88–92
Alzheimer's disease, 82–84
Ama, 25
Apa, 25
Apana, 25
American diet, 216
Antioxidants, 50, 267, 273
Aromatherapy, 17
Arthritis, 60–68, 254
Artificial sweeteners, 183
Asana, 25
Atharva veda, 26
Attaining longevity, 4
Ayurveda, 23–31
Bali, 26
Beta carotene, 273
Biblical Diet, 218
Bland Diet, 220
Body for Life Diet, 236
Brain, aging, 57–60
Calcium, 27, 190, 214
Calories, 223
Cancer, 115–120, 241
Carbohydrates, 183,213
Chakra, 426
Chinese Diet, 226
Cholesterol, 131
Chronic fatigue, 69
Complimentary therapies, 13
Constipation, 78
Decoction, 26
Depression 73–74
Dehydration, 104–107, 288
Dermatix, 56
Dhatu, 45

Diabetes, 185, 204
Diets, 200
Dinacharya, 27
Doshas, 27
Emesis, 27
Exercise, 11, 215, 280
Faith healing, 147
Fast food, 251
Fat(s), 78, 155, 203
Fertility, 135
Fiber, 9, 214
Fibromyalgia, 69
Flower remedies, 196
Flu shots, 139
Flu prevention, 144
Folic acid, 10
Food chain, 6
Foods, healing, 162–170
French Diet, 244
French Thalo therapy, 53
Free radicals, 162, 267
Fruits, 268
Gallstones, 77
Gandharva, 27
Ghee, 27
Gluten, wheat, 179
Guna, 28
Health, how to, 7–12, 154
Health, transformation, 1
Hearing, 47
Heat Illness, (see Dehydration)
Heart Health, 121–152,265
Heart Disease Diet, 121, 242
Heart Testing, 129–132
Herbs, healing, 189
Homeopathy, 18–21
Hypoglycemia, 76
Iron, 10
Influenza, 142
Jala, 27

Japanese Diet, 221
Karma, 27
Katu, 27
Kidneys, 49
Liposuction, 108
Liver, 49, 84–87, 254
Maha Bhutas, 28
Magnesium, 271
Marma, 28
Massage, 112
Meat (red), 174, 203, 227
Medications, 47
Meditation, 32–37
Mediterranean Diet, 230
Metabolic rate, 285
Metabolic syndrome, 133–134
Mosquito Borne Disease, 96–100
Motion sickness, 92
Muscle aches, 51
Nadi, 28
Natriuretic peptides, 131
Nutrition, 185, 219
Nuts, 179–183
Obesity, 252
Ojas, 28
Omega-3 Fatty acids, 9
Ornish Diet, 238
Panchakarma, 28
Pitta, 28
Portfolio Diet, 234
Pragnyaparadha, 29
Prakriti, 29
Pranayama, 29
Purgation, 29
Purification, 47
Quantum, 30
Rajas, 30
Rasas, 30
Rasayana, 30
Recipes, 291–330

Reiki, 21
Rejuventation, 18
Respiratory, 254
Rishi, 30
SAD Diet, 200
Satva, 30
Scarprin, 56
Seer, 30
Sugar alcohols, 184
Senses, 44
Shiatsu, 22
Sleep disorders, 73
Soy, 177
Stroke, 244, 254
Stress, 74, 139
Surgery, 107
Surya Namaskara, 30
Tamas, 30
Tattoos, 94–96
Tempeh, 179
Thallotherapy, 278
Theraeutic massage, 109
Tofu, 177
Transformational medicine, 153
Travel Tips, 103
Vaccinations, 101, 161
Vata, 31
Vedic, 31
Vegan Diet, 170
Vegetarian Diet, 240
Vegetables, 275
Vision, 44
Vitamins, 189, 275
Water, 158
Weight Loss, 257
Weil's Diet, 248
Wrinkles 54, 161
Yoga, 31
Yogic, 31
Zinc, 111, 190, 198

PAUL DAVIS MD

BABY BOOMER LONGEVITY

STRATEGIES TO TRANSFORM YOUR HEALTH

Paul Davis MD is also the author of *Cruise Ship Crime Mysteries: A Medical Murder Mystery, The Curious Cargo of Bones and The German Intrigue.* He was trained in Family Practice and Emergency Medicine in Canada, the United Kingdom and the United States. Dr. Davis uses his insider knowledge, as his novels are based on his ten-year career as a cruise ship doctor. He currently lives in Canada and is the director of a medical specialty group.

http://www.cruiseshipcrimesite.com
http://cruiseshipcrime.wordpress.com

Dr. Paul Davis is available for lectures and readings. For information regarding his availability, please contact Skye Wentworth, Publicist at 978-462-4453 or email skyewentworth@gmail.com.

January 2013

www.ingramcontent.com/pod-product-compliance
Lightning Source LLC
Chambersburg PA
CBHW082129290526

45794CB00008B/2973